Diagnosis and Treatment
of Functional Infertility

B. Lunenfeld, V. Insler, M. Glezerman

Bruno Lunenfeld
Vaclav Insler
Marek Glezerman

Diagnosis and Treatment of Functional Infertility

3rd revised edition
Preface by E. E. Wallach

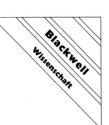

Blackwell Wissenschaft · Berlin 1993

Bruno Lunenfeld, MD, FRCOG, Professor of Life Sciences, Bar Ilan University; Ramat Gan, Israel.

Vaclav Insler, MD, FRCOG, Professor of Obstetrics and Gynecology, Hebrew University, Hadassah Medical School; Director, Department of Obstetrics & Gynecology, Kaplan Hospital, Rehovoth, Israel.

Marek Glezerman, MD, Professor of Obstetrics and Gynecology, Faculty of Health Sciences, Ben-Gurion University of the Negev; Chairman, Departments of Obstetrics & Gynecology, Soroka Medical Center, Beer-Sheba, Israel.

ISBN 3-89412-129-7

Die Deutsche Bibliothek – CIP-Einheitsaufnahme

Lunenfeld, Bruno:
Diagnosis and treatment of functional infertility / Bruno Lunenfeld; Vaclav Insler; Marek Glezerman.
Pref. by E. E. Wallach. – (3., rev. ed.). – Berlin: Blackwell-Wiss.-Verl., 1992
  ISBN 3-89412-129-7
NE: Insler, Vaclav:; Glezerman, Marek:

© Blackwell Wissenschafts-Verlag GmbH Berlin 1992
Printed in Germany

The citing of proprietary names, trade names, product descriptions, etc, in this work, even where not specially designated, does not justify the assumption that such names can be regarded as disposable within the meaning of the trade marks and trade marks protection legislation and therefore open to be used by anyone.
Product liability: The publishers can accept no liability for details of dosage instructions and presentations. The accuracy of details of this sort should be checked by the respective user in each individual case using other reference sources.

Cover design: R. Hübler, Berlin
Typesetting: Acron Verlag GmbH, Berlin
Printing and binding: ProPrint Druck- und Verlags oHG, Berlin

To our families

PREFACE

The field of infertility has undergone dramatic change over the past 15 years. The challenges in providing care to the infertile couple have traditionally been related to the step-wise analysis of individual factors which may be interfering with a given couple's ability to establish a pregnancy and the use of medical and surgical means to correct their impediments to conception. The advent of the era of in vitro fertilization which began in 1978 with the birth of Louise Brown has altered the traditional approach considerably, permitting the entrance into the field of infertility of a unique style of infertility specialist interested in the new procedurally oriented technologies, which include endoscopic surgical procedures and in vitro fertilization and its offshoots. Unfortunately the wide scale use of the latter technology as a panacea for infertility due to a wide range of putative causes or for infertility which goes unexplained tends to reduce the analytical and logical evaluation and management which has typified the field in the past. It will also retard new developments in management of certain aspects of infertility.

For this reason, as well as for many others, this textbook by Lunenfeld, Insler and Glezerman is a refreshing addition to the library of the serious practitioner involved in the care of infertile couples. The allusion to IVF and related technologies is minimal. Instead the authors have divided their text into an almost equal page distribution between female and male infertility. Following a concise and lucid discussion of physiologic principles governing folliculogenesis, spermatogenesis and hormonal elaboration in male and female, the authors logically review in a step-wise manner conditions in which components vital to normal reproduction are dysfunctional. They then proceed to analyze each alternative. For example, the spectrum of pharmacologic agents available for ovulation induction are reviewed, as well as virtues and drawbacks of each. The statistics presented represent broad input from various groups and are not restricted to the statistics generated by the three authors themselves.

Equally refreshing is that in an era of multi-authored textbooks, three distinguished figures in the field of infertility have combined their enormous experience in producing a text which is easily readable, not redundant, and reflects a philosophy based upon extensive personal experience. Few textbooks today send themselves to cover to cover reading. **Diagnosis and Treatment of Functional Infertility** represents just such a text. It will not only benefit the readers, but their infertile couples will also be aided in accomplishing their goals of maximizing their childbearing potential.

Edward E. Wallach, M.D.

CONTENTS

Female Infertility

1. INTRODUCTION

The periodic maturation and discharge of a fertilizable egg is the cornerstone of the female reproductive process. This event is accompanied by profound organic, functional and behavioral changes throughout the entire individual. The rhythm of these changes determines to a large extent the nature of the adult life of a female in a simple rodent, in the primate, and, in fact, in the human. The ovulatory cycle is governed and accompanied by characteristic protein and hormonal levels that are reflected in typical changes in the reproductive organs. To enable grouping, superimposition, recording, and comparison of various parameters of the ovulatory cycle, its span is divided into several phases. Each phase reflects a characteristic, easily definable hormonal or organic change. Depending on the criteria on which the division is based, several different phases of the ovulatory cycle may be recognized. In the following discussion the simple division into follicular, ovulatory and luteal phases will be used (Fig. 1–1).

The follicular phase actually begins 4 to 5 days before menstrual bleeding and lasts until the appearance of the midcycle LH surge, encompassing the periods of follicular recruitment (rescue), selection of the dominant follicle, its developmental growth, and maturation. It is characterized by elevated levels of FSH and low levels of LH, estrogens, and progesterone during the recruitment and selection phases. This is followed by an increase of estrogens during the growth and maturation of the dominant follicle. The ovulatory phase is characterized by the estrogen-evoked LH surge, followed by a decline in estrogen levels and a rise in progesterone levels. This is accompanied by the resumption of the first meiotic division by the oocyte, rupture of the follicle, and extrusion of the egg.

The post-ovulatory or luteal phase is characterized by a marked rise in progesterone levels, which reach a plateau about five days after ovulation. Concomitant with the rise in progesterone levels, the basal body temperature (BBT) rises. The association of estrogen and progesterone prepares the uterus for implantation of the fertilized egg and inhibits FSH and LH secretion via negative feedback control at the hypothalamic and pituitary level. FSH and LH remain low during the luteal phase. If ovulation is followed by fertilization and conception, then by the ninth post-ovulatory day, hCG appears in the circulation. Its rapid rise prevents corpus luteum regression and stimulates corpus luteum function as expressed in a further increase in both estrogens and progesterone. In the absence of conception, the corpus luteum regresses and estrogen and progesterone levels decline around the tenth day following ovulation. This marks the beginning of the late luteal (premenstrual) phase. The declining levels of estrogens and progesterone cause endometrial shedding (menstruation) and provoke the increase of FSH which marks the beginning of follicular recruitment of the following cycle.

Fig. 1–1. Human menstrual cycle. Schematic presentation of hormonal profiles and ovarian and endometrial events.   ▶

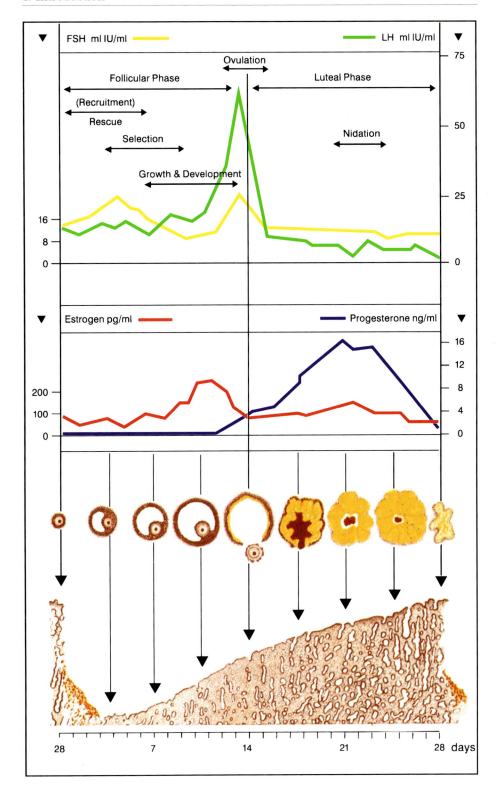

2. REGULATION OF THE FEMALE REPRODUCTIVE SYSTEM

Sensory stimuli from the external environment, such as visual and olfactory stimuli, stress, as well as internal stimuli, cause brain nerve fibers to release neurotransmitters, i.e., catecholamines, indolamines, and cholinergic agents (Fig. 2–1). These neuro-transmitters regulate the pulsatile secretion of gonadotropin-releasing hormone(s) (GnRH) from neurosecretory cells located mainly in the arcuate nucleus of the hypothalamus (Kamberi, 1975; Knobil, 1980).

It appears that under the proper steroid environment, catecholamines (dopamine, norepinephrine, or epinephrine) and the cholinergic agent acetylcholine exert a stimulating influence on the pulsatile secretory pattern of GnRH, whereas endorphines and indolamines (serotonin or its metabolic product melatonin) have an opposite effect. In turn, pulses of GnRH of a specific amplitude and frequency reach the anterior pituitary via the hypophyseal portal system and control gonadotropin secretion.

The gonadotropins are synthesized in the oval basophil cells of the adenohypophy-sis and, evidently, both gonadotropins originate in the same type of cell. A simple mechanism in which a single releasing hormone (GnRH) regulates secretion of both gonadotropic hormones would be insufficient to account for the fluctuations in the ratio of FSH to LH secretion observed during the menstrual cycle and in various pathological states. Cyclic fluctuations in the FSH/LH ratio are achieved by a differential sensitivity of the pituitary to GnRH under the influence of sex steroids.

The next message in this molecular relay is conveyed by means of FSH and LH. FSH binds almost exclusively to membrane receptors on the granulosa cells, induces their multiplication, and stimulates biochemical processes such as aromatase activity, while LH stimulates theca cell development and androgen production. Androgens diffusing into the granulosa cell layer are converted to estrogens. FSH together with estrogens induce synthesis of FSH and LH receptors on the granulosa cells, leading to increased sensitivity of the growing follicle to gonadotropins.

The first step in the action of gonadotropins on the ovary is their binding to specific receptor sites on the plasma membrane of ovarian cells (Channing and Kammerman, 1974).

FSH binds almost exclusively to granulosa cells, while LH binds primarily to thecal cells and corpus luteum tissue. The initial binding of gonadotropins to receptor sites is followed by activation of a membrane-localized adenylate cyclase system, thereby resulting in an increase of intracellular levels of cAMP. In turn, cAMP – the second messenger – mediates hormonal induction of ovarian RNA and activates the protein system necessary for ovum maturation and steroidogenesis (Jungmann et al. 1974; Tsafriri et al. 1973; Younglai, 1975).

During the last few years, the importance of intraovarian regulation via the potentiating effect of growth hormone releasing hormone (GRF), growth hormone (GH), an array of different growth factors, and insulin on both the thecal cell response to LH and the granulosa cell response to FSH has been demonstrated (Adashi et al. 1985; Barbieri et al. 1988; Blumenfeld and Lunenfeld, 1989).

Steroid hormones produced by the ovary fulfill several functions:

1. They regulate follicular maturation by intraovarian mechanism(s);
2. they provide the proper hormonal milieu in the reproductive

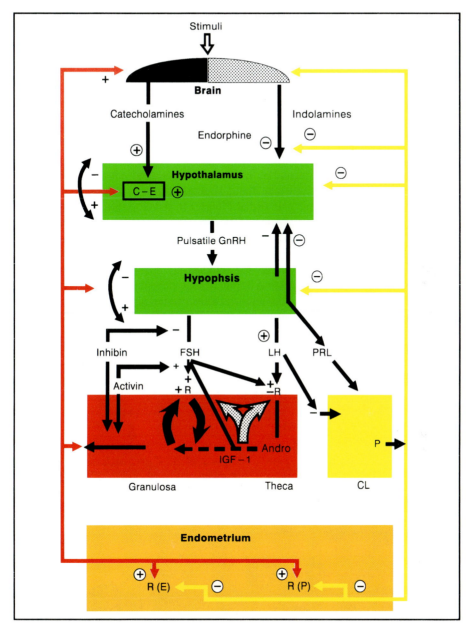

Fig. 2-1. Regulatory mechanisms of ovarian function.
The control of the function of ovarian compartments such as granulosa, theca, and corpus luteum (CL) is accomplished through three different mechanisms:
1. Stimulation along the brain-hypothalamus-hypophysis-ovarian axis by neurotransmitters (C–E = catecholestrogens), pulsatile GnRH, FSH, LH, and prolactin (PRL).
2. Intraovarian modulation of hormone receptors (R) by the positive influence of FSH and estrogens (E-2) and the negative influence of androgens (Andro). Insulin-like growth factor (IGF-1) enhances FSH-stimulated granulosa cells differentiation and epidermal growth factors (EGF) modulate cell differentiation.
3. Feedback signals, positive (+) and negative (-), by ovarian estrogens, progesterone (P), inhibin and activin.

organs for the transport of gametes and sustaining nidation of the fertilized
ovum;
3. they modulate FSH and LH secretion via feedback control at the hypothalamic
and pituitary levels.

FOLLICULAR DEVELOPMENT

Early studies based on animal experiments suggested that follicular development up
to the antrum stage was gonadotropin-independent. Lunenfeld and Eshkol (1967)
showed that in prepubertal mice deprived of gonadotropin, follicular development
could proceed; however, it was markedly altered and retarded. Gougeon (1985) has
suggested that, in women, it may take about 10 weeks for an oocyte surrounded by a
single layer of granulosa cells (primordial follicle) to develop into an antral follicle
capable of gonadotropic responsiveness. Final growth, maturation and ovulation will
then occur within two weeks under optimal FSH and LH stimulation and normal
ovarian response. Whereas several hundred primordial follicles probably start to
grow, no more than about 20 precursor follicles are likely to be present at the
beginning of the menstrual cycle. All the others degenerate at early stages of
development. Of about twenty remaining follicles, under physiological conditions,
some will be selected for further growth and development, but only one will mature,
reach dominance, and ovulate. The others will undergo atresia, or luteinization
(Fig. 2-2).

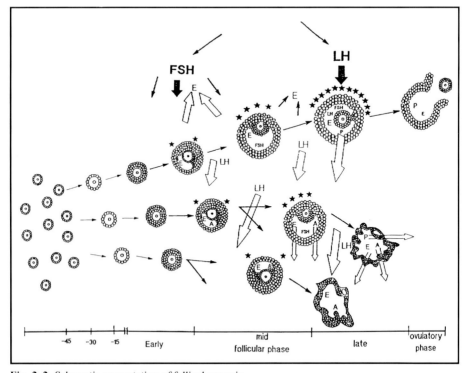

Fig. 2-2. Schematic presentation of folliculogenesis.
The upper row shows folliculogenesis leading to ovulation, the middle row to luteinization, and the
lower row to atresia. * = receptors, E = estrogens, A = androgens, P = progesterone

According to Hodgen and his coworkers (Goodman et al. 1977; Hodgen, 1982), in the primate model the gonadotropin-dependent folliculogenesis proceeds by the following steps:

1. Recruitment of a follicular cohort is dependent on the rise of FSH levels which takes place 4–5 days before the onset of menstrual bleeding (Ross et al. 1970; Landgren et al. 1980).
2. Selection from the recruited follicular cohort of a follicle destined to reach the state of dominance and subsequently ovulate. The selection process is completed during the early follicular phase (usually within the first seven days of the cycle).
3. Follicular dominance. Following its selection, the dominant follicle grows and matures at a higher rate than the other follicles due to its increased sensitivity to FSH. Moreover, by producing estrogen as well as inhibin the dominant follicle regulates gonadotropin secretion, which enables its final maturation on the one hand and inhibits further development of other follicles of the same cohort on the other hand.
4. At the proper time, the dominant follicle causes the occurrence of the estrogen-provoked LH surge and subsequently ovulates and is transformed into a functional corpus luteum.

While the actions of pituitary gonadotropins have been well characterized, the role of growth hormone (GH) in ovarian function has only recently been discovered. GH administered to hypophysectomized female rats increases the in vitro steroidogenic responsiveness to FSH, whereas reduction of serum growth hormone in intact rats reduces ovarian responsiveness to gonadotrophins. The fact that GH-dependent local production of insulin-like growth factor (IGF-1) can directly enhance FSH-stimulated ovarian granulosa cell differentiation may indicate the existence of a novel paracrine or autocrine mechanism by which ovarian development can be controlled (Jia et al. 1985; Adashi et al. 1985). It is of interest to note that, in 1972, Sheikholislam & Stempfel already observed that growth hormone therapy could advance puberty in patients with delayed puberty associated with isolated GH deficiency.

Given the pivotal role of FSH in the induction of its own granulosa cell receptors as well as those for LH and possibly beta2–adrenergic ligands, the demonstration of FSH-enhanced somatomedin C (SmC) binding strongly suggests that the acquisition of SmC (IGF-1) responsiveness may be part and parcel of granulosa cell ontogeny. Accordingly, enhancement of SmC binding may be a mechanism whereby gonadotropins may condition the cell to respond optimally to SmC, thereby conferring a selective advantage upon follicles so endowed. It is thus tempting to speculate that the granulosa cell SmC receptor complement may constitute one of several variables responsible for follicular selection and the assertion of follicular dominance.

Intraovarian Regulation by Steroids

Ovarian production of estrogen brings about follicular maturation by increasing follicular sensitivity to gonadotropin stimulation through the following sequential mechanism: Alone or together with FSH, estrogen induces synthesis of ovarian FSH receptors, which leads to increased FSH binding and a consequent stimulation of ovarian LH receptors (Channing and Tsafriri, 1974; Louvet and Vaitukaitis, 1975; Richards and Midgley, 1976). Androgens, on the other hand, inhibit the synthesis of both FSH and LH receptors. It may be speculated that the cAMP inhibitor present in follicular fluid (Channing and Tsafriri, 1974; Kraiem and Lunenfeld, 1978) might interfere with luteinization and oocyte maturation (Channing and Tsafriri, 1974). Follicular fluid constituents, analogous to male inhibin, modulate the secretion of FSH and may also influence FSH action at the ovarian level. Regarding intraovarian mechanism(s) involving progesterone, it has been suggested (Rondell, 1974) that the secretion of this steroid by thecal cells stimulates an ovulatory enzyme (plasmin ?) (Beers et al. 1975) which, by proteolytic action, causes a distortion of the collagen framework of the follicular wall. Concomitantly, a rise in prostaglandins takes place (Bauminger and Lindner, 1975). Follicular rupture and ovum extrusion may thus be regarded as a consequence of several interacting effects: the diminished stretchability of the follicular wall and the prostaglandin-induced contraction of the muscular elements of the follicular wall. While some follicles grow to full maturity and ovulate, many more undergo atresia.

Atresia may be promoted by the local effect of ovarian androgens (Speroff and Van-de Wiele, 1971; Louvet et al. 1975). The ovaries of immature rats contain abundant 5-alpha reductase activity (Armstrong et al. 1975) and have been reported to secrete substantial amounts of 5-alpha-reduced androgens (Eckstein and Ravard, 1974). It is conceivable that one of these compounds might cause atresia. Consistent with this possibility are reports that dihydrotestosterone (DHT) and 5-alpha-androstane-3,17-dione are effective inhibitors of aromatase (Schwarzel et al. 1973).

Estrogens have been shown both to prevent atresia and to promote growth of preantral follicles. It has been shown (Armstrong and Papkoff, 1976) that LH stimulates ovarian androgen production by theca interna cells whereas FSH enhances granulosa cell conversion of androgens to 17–beta estradiol by inducing aromatase activity. Thus, the fate of each follicle is essentially determined by a delicate interplay between:

1. the relative amounts of LH and FSH available
2. the relative amounts of FSH and LH bound to follicular receptors
3. the relative amounts of estrogens and androgens.

A follicle capable of binding FSH and LH in the proper amounts and sequence will produce enough intrafollicular estrogens to mature and ovulate. On the other hand, a follicle incapable of binding enough FSH or receiving too much LH will synthesize mainly androgen and will be doomed to atresia. Thus, the 2 types of testosterone metabolites, estrogen and 5-alpha reduced androgens, exert opposing actions upon the follicles – estrogens leading to ovulation and androgens to atresia.

Effect of Steroids on Uterine Function

Ovarian steroids regulate endometrial growth and development. The frequency of endometrial mitoses during the follicular phase of the primate cycle can be directly correlated with the action of estrogens. Today it is well established that estradiol enters into the endometrial cells and binds noncovalently to the estrogen acceptor molecule. This is followed by conformational changes resulting in the formation of a hormone-receptor complex. This complex associates with chromatin (DNA) components of the nucleus and elicits the normal event of expression, i.e. messenger RNA formation, transcription, processing, and translation. The above chain of events will result in the biological activity of the estrogen target cell. In the endometrial cell, it will evoke mitotic activity, cell differentiation, and synthesis of various proteins including enzymes and estrogen and progesterone receptors. Thus, estrogen regulates its own receptor synthesis by a feedback mechanism. Progesterone binds to the estrogen-induced progesterone acceptor. Following the formation of the progesterone-receptor complex and its binding to the cell nucleus, a specific chain of biological events will be induced. This includes inhibition of mitotic activity, inhibition of receptors for both estrogen and progesterone, as well as structural and functional changes in the cell, resulting in the transformation of proliferative into secretory endometrium. These changes are crucial for preparing the endometrium for the nidation of a fertilized egg. It may be speculated that the effect of estradiol upon the endometrium depends on two elements: the absolute level of the hormone and the duration of its action.

On the other hand, the effect of progesterone depends on prior estrogenic stimulation and also on the estrogen/progesterone ratio. Thus, the greater the estrogen-induced endometrial tissue mass, the more progesterone will be necessary in order to result in its secretory transformation and function.

The maintenance of secretory endometrium requires continuous estrogen and progesterone stimulation. Thus, regression of corpus luteum function, resulting in a decrease in steroid levels, will evoke endometrial shedding accompanied by uterine bleeding. On the other hand, the rescue of the corpus luteum by hCG and other factors secreted by the trophoblast will maintain the endometrial integrity and function. During the secretory phase of the cycle and in early pregnancy, the endometrium is more sensitive to the pattern of estrogen and progesterone secretion and their ratio than to the absolute levels of these hormones.

It should be noted that steroid hormones influence the structure and function of the endometrium not only on the cellular but also on the whole organ level (Kleinman et al. 1983). This is especially due to the hormonal action upon the blood vessels. The size and functional integrity of spiral arteries is of primary importance to the biological function of the endometrium. It should be noted that the main uterine and spiral arteries contain estrogen receptors and thus their anatomy and function is to a large extent dependent on this hormone. If, however, the functional layer of the endometrium is stimulated by estrogen to increase its thickness more than the concomitant stimulation of spiral arteries evokes their elongation, the uppermost layer of the endometrium may not receive a sufficient blood supply. The consequence of this situation is the occurrence of break-through bleeding.

ROLE OF STEROIDS IN FEEDBACK CONTROL OF GONADOTROPHIN SECRETION

The central role of ovarian steroids in the feedback modulation of gonadotrophic secretion is well established (Speroff and Vande Wiele, 1971). Metaphorically speaking, as colorfully depicted by Short, the hypothalamus and pituitary appear to dance to a tune played upon them by the ovarian steroids (Short, 1974). Steroids exert a dual feedback action upon gonadotrophic secretion, having both negative inhibitory and positive stimulatory effects. It is well known that increasing amounts of estradiol as well as a combination of estrogens and progesterone inhibit the secretion of gonadotrophins. The special feature of this regulating mechanism is the ability of estrogens to provoke a midcycle gonadotrophin surge. It may be speculated that this surge is brought about by the following sequence of events:

1. The estradiol rising during the late follicular phase does not significantly change the pulsatile pattern of GnRH secretion.

2. In a predominantly estrogenic milieu, the pituitary gland produces more LH than FSH, thus increasing the amount of LH produced by the gonadotrophs.
3. Because of the inhibitory effect of rising estrogen levels (and other follicle-produced inhibitory material, e.g. inhibin) on the ability of the pituitary gland to release gonadotropins, the amount of gonadotropins (predominantly LH) stored in the hypophysis rises.
4. When the storage of gonadotropins reaches a certain threshold (72–140 hrs following the exponential rise in estrogens) the entire gonadotropin reservoir is released.

This is due either to the decrease of estrogens, intrafollicular inhibitory proteins, or the storage capacity of the pituitary. This results in the midcycle LH surge and FSH rise. It is the midcycle preovulatory surge of gonadotropins which leads to the final steps of follicular maturation (Channing and Tsafriri, 1974; Kraiem and Lunenfeld, 1978). This surge effects the resumption of oocyte meiosis and ovulation by overcoming the inhibitory influence exerted by the follicular fluid. The surge of gonadotropins itself is triggered by estrogen alone, though in some species the mechanism also requires synergistic action of progestogens (Speroff and Vande Wiele, 1971; Swerdloff et al. 1972). The shutoff mechanism of the LH surge may operate through a shortloop feedback mechanism. Hypothalamic and pituitary cystine arylamidase, which inactivates GnRH, has been shown to be stimulated by LH acting synergistically with sex steroids (Kuhl and Taubert, 1975, 1975a). Finally, gonadal steroids also appear to regulate gonadotropic secretion by modulating, at the pituitary level, gonadotropic response to the GnRH stimulus (Eshkol et al. 1975).

It has been suggested by several investigators (Bogdanove, 1964; Docke and Dorner, 1965; Davidson, 1969; Arimura and Schally, 1970) that, in addition to their action on the hypothalamus, gonadal steroids might also exert a direct effect on the pituitary gland.

Hilliard, Schally and Sawyer (1971) found that pituitary implants of progesterone prevented GnRH-induced LH release in rabbits. Arimura and Schally (1970) found that pretreatment of rats with progesterone blocked, at least partially, the LH release induced by GnRH. Dierschke et al. (1973) also found that progesterone blocked the positive feedback action of estrogen on LH release in the rhesus monkey, and postulated that progesterone acts at centers higher than the pituitary.

The various experimental approaches and interpretations of the results cited above are based on systems in which both the pituitary gland and the hypothalamus were involved. In order to elucidate the action of steroids on the pituitary, hypothalamic influences had to be eliminated. To do this, the effect of releasing hormone was studied in patients with primary hypothalamic amenorrhea and apparently normal pituitary ovarian axis under different steroidal environments (Lunenfeld et al. 1974).

In the presence of low endogenous estrogen and progesterone levels (compatible with the early follicular phase of a normal ovulatory cycle), the administration of GnRH resulted in a significant rise of both FSH and LH.

In the presence of high estrogen and low progesterone levels (compatible with the preovulatory phase of the normal cycle), the administration of GnRH caused a diminished FSH response and an exaggerated LH secretion.

The administration of GnRH in the presence of high estrogen and elevated progesterone levels (compatible with the luteal phase of a normal cycle) evoked only a relatively small release of either FSH or LH.

Therefore, it can be postulated that steroids, by selectively modifying pituitary responsiveness, can cause the preferential release of either FSH or LH, resulting in varying FSH/LH ratios secreted in response to the same stimulant. It has been well demonstrated that prolactin, if secreted in excess, can cause anovulation or luteal insufficiency. It seems that in contrast to its effect on rodents, where it stimulates luteal function, in the human, prolactin affects the frequency and amplitude of GnRH pulsatility and thus deranges the normal pattern of gonadotropin secretion, resulting in disorderly follicular development.

Any disruption in the delicately coordinated interaction between the integrated components of the hypothalamic-pituitary-ovarian axis, which must operate within precise quantitative limits and accurate temporal sequences, may lead to anovulation. The above outlined advances in reproductive endocrinology have led to a better understanding of the basic mechanisms regulating these processes and governing reproductive function. This has furnished the impetus for transforming the field of female infertility from a largely empirical venture to the firmer ground of a more rational approach.

3. CLASSIFICATION OF ANOVULATORY STATES

Roughly one third of the infertile population seeking advice at infertility clinics show ovulation failure. Anovulation may be accompanied by a variety of menstrual disorders, the nature of which is directly related to the level and type of fluctuation of the ovarian steroids. Several cycle-regulating and ovulation-inducing drugs are available and each of them may be used at various dosage levels or treatment schemes. A decision has to be made as to the type of therapy each patient should receive. The treatment will be reasonably successful and safe only if this decision is correct. In other words, proper classification of patients is a *sine qua non* for effective and safe therapy. Moreover, comparison of the results obtained in various groups of patients at the same center or of patients treated at different centers is possible only if a well-defined and reproducible classification has been used. The possibilities for classifying anovulatory patients are virtually unlimited, depending on the clinical and laboratory facilities available and the purpose to be served. Every classification may be valuable as long as acceptable measurable and well-defined parameters are used, and as long as a reasonable compromise is achieved between the accuracy, effort, and cost required. It should also be noted that the constant development of new drugs, the widening scope of knowledge regarding the physiology and endocrinology of the reproductive processes, as well as the rapid development of new diagnostic methods and therapeutic procedures, necessitates the continuous reassessment and updating of ramifications of the classification system without changing its basic philosophy (Table 3-1).

Needless to say, a complete fertility survey including evaluation of the mechanical, male, immunological, and cervical factors must be carried out in each case before treatment is initiated.

In the early sixties, when only gonadotrophins and clomiphene citrate were available, our group used a simple therapeutically-oriented classification (Insler et al. 1968) which has been modified and adopted by the WHO Scientific Group (World Health Organization, Technical Report Series, 1973). With this classification, patients were divided into 3 main groups:

Group I
Women with primary or secondary amenorrhea, low levels of endogenous gonadotrophins, and negligible endogenous estrogen activity (urinary estrogens usually less than 10 mcg/24 hrs).

Group II
Patients with anovulation associated with a variety of menstrual disorders (including amenorrhea) who exhibit distinct endogenous estrogen activity (urinary estrogens usually more than 10 mcg/24 hrs) and whose urinary and serum gonadotrophins are in the normal range.

Group III
Women with primary or secondary amenorrhea due to primary ovarian failure associated with low endogenous estrogen activity and pathologically high gonadotrophin levels.

TABLE 3–1. Stages leading to the Development of therapeutically oriented Classification of anovulatory States

1955	*Clinical use of urinary hormone assays (steroids and gonadotropins)*
1959	*Availability of hPG, hMG, and hCG for clinical research*
1960	Attempt at classification of patients suitable for gonadotrophic therapy
1961	*Introduction of clomiphene citrate for clinical research*
1965	Wide-scale clinical use of clomiphene citrate and gonadotropins
1968	*Introduction of progesterone challenge test*
1968	**FIRST THERAPEUTICALLY ORIENTED CLASSIFICATION (4 GROUPS)**
1970	*Routine use of radio-immuno-assays*
1970	*Availability of native GnRH for clinical testing*
1972	Introduction of prolactin assays
1974	Introduction of prolactin-inhibiting agents
1976	**SECOND THERAPEUTICALLY ORIENTED CLASSIFICATION (7 GROUPS)**
1979	*Application of ultrasound in the examination of ovarian follicles*
1980	Introduction of pulsatile GnRH therapy
1982	Introduction of purified FSH for clinical use
1985	The use of GnRH analogs combined with gonadotropins in ovulation-induction protocols
1988	**PRESENT CLASSIFICATION (10 GROUPS)**
1992	Introduction of FSH by recombinant DNA technology

However, scientific and technical advances made during the next few years, i.e., the discovery of the effect of hyperprolactinemia on the reproductive function and on the availability of prolactin-inhibiting agents, required the introduction of a corresponding modification in the classification of patients receiving ovulation-inducing therapy. Such a modification was introduced in 1976 (WHO Scientific Group Meeting, Hamburg, 1976), and the classification was enlarged to 7 groups:

Group I
Hypothalamic-Pituitary Failure-amenorrheic women with no evidence of endogenous estrogen production, with non-elevated prolactin levels, with normal or low FSH levels and no detectable space-occupying lesion in the hypothalamic pituitary region.

Group II
Hypothalamic-Pituitary Dysfunction-women with a variety of menstrual cycle disturbances, e.g. luteal phase insufficiency, anovulatory cycles, and amenorrhea with evidence of endogenous estrogen production and normal prolactin and FSH levels.

Group III
Ovarian Failure – amenorrheic women with no evidence of ovarian estrogen production and with elevated FSH levels but non-elevated prolactin levels.

Group IV
Congenital or Acquired Genital Tract Disorder-amenorrheic women who do not respond to repeated administrations of estrogen with withdrawal bleeding.

Group V
Hyperprolactinemic Infertile Women with a Space-Occupying Lesion in the Hypothalamic-Pituitary Region – women with a variety of menstrual cycle disturbances, e.g. luteal phase insufficiency, anovulatory cycles, or amenorrhea, with elevated prolactin levels and evidence of a space-occupying lesion in the hypothalamic-pituitary region.

Group VI
Hyperprolactinemic Infertile Women with No Detectable Space-Occupying Lesion in the Hypothalamic-Pituitary Region – the same as Group V women except that there is no evidence of a space-occupying lesion.

Group VII
Amenorrheic Women with Non-Elevated Prolactin Levels and Evidence of a Space-Occupying Lesion in the Hypothalamic-Pituitary Region – women with low endogenous estrogen production and normal or low prolactin and FSH levels.

This classification hinged mainly upon 3 parameters, the levels of endogenous prolactin, gonadotropins, and estrogens. Gonadotropins in the urine may be estimated as the total gonadotropic activity or, preferably, by specific assay of serum follicle stimulating hormone (FSH) and luteinizing hormone (LH). It would be difficult to specify absolute FSH and LH levels as uniquely characteristic for each of the 3 groups. However, a rough distinction between low, normal, and high (menopausal) gonadotropin levels should not present a complicated problem, regardless of the method and type of standard preparation used. The extent of endogenous estrogen activity can be estimated either by direct measurement of urinary or plasma estrogens, or by indirect methods such as cervical score endometrial biopsy (Noyes, 1966) and the occurrence or lack of uterine bleeding after administration of progesterone or a progesterone-like compound (progesterone challenge test).

Practically, the division of patients into the aforementioned groups was carried out as follows: Women with hyperprolactinemia, regardless of the type of their menstrual cyclicity, were classified under Group V, when a space-occupying lesion of the hypothalamic-pituitary region was identifiable, and under Group VI when such a lesion was not present. Normoprolactinemic patients could then be further classified as spontaneous bleeders or amenorrheic.

Spontaneous bleeders and amenorrheic patients responding to administration of a progestational compound with withdrawal bleeding were classified under Group II (Hypothalamic-pituitary dysfunction). The occurrence of spontaneous bleeding, however irregular, or withdrawal bleeding after progesterone indicates 5 important findings:

1. the presence of a uterus with endometrium capable of normal response to ovarian steroids.
2. The presence of some endogenous estrogen activity which, in turn, indicates:
3. the presence of at least minimal ovarian activity
4. the presence of gonadotropic stimulation sufficient to evoke follicular maturation (probably beyond antrum stage)
5. the presence of hypothalamic GnRH activity sufficient for basic pituitary stimulation.

It is conceivable that a situation may arise when all the main components of the hypothalamic-hypophyseal-ovarian system are capable of function, but the feedback mechanism regulating the overall activity is malfunctioning.

If, after administration of the gestagen, withdrawal bleeding did not occur, sequential treatment with estrogen and progesterone was given. A positive response, i.e. uterine bleeding, indicated that a uterus capable of response was present but the ovaries did not provide the required steroids. At this stage, estimation of urinary or plasma gonadotropins had to be carried out in order to distinguish between pituitary and ovarian failure. High gonadotropin levels (menopausal values) indicated the ovaries as the cause of amenorrhea (Group III). Chromosomal studies and ovarian biopsy through the laparoscope might then be performed. A pathological karyotype (XO, XY, or mosaic) or ovarian histology showing a complete lack of follicles (Black & Govan, 1972) would indicate that any attempt at stimulating ovarian activity would be fruitless. Low or undetectable gonadotropins indicated hypothalamic-pituitary failure (Group I). Finally, those patients who did not show uterine bleeding after administration of estrogen and progesterone had to be considered. In these, pregnancy, traumatic or inflammatory lesions of the uterus or cervix (Asherman's Syndrome), and congenital malformations of the genital tract such as absence of uterus, vaginal atresia, or imperforate hymen should be ruled out by appropriate examination (Group IV).

The above-mentioned classification has been simple enough to be applied to a large number of patients and accurate enough to enable the choice of the ovulation-inducing agents then available. It has also been proven to be effective in assessing the prognosis of the treatment and comparing the results obtained.

Within the last decade, new knowledge regarding the physiology of ovulation has emerged, diagnostic and monitoring techniques have been refined, and new therapeutic agents were introduced. Furthermore the experience obtained by large-scale clinical application of this classification indicated the need for introducing additional changes.

Experience has indicated that nonfunctional pituitary tumors are extremely rare in infertile women. Thus, Group VII has been excluded from the present classification.

The availability of pulsatile GnRH treatment required a subdivision of Group I into hypothalamic and pituitary failure by means of a GnRH test (see Chapter 4). In both subgroups, gonadotropin therapy is highly effective, while in the responders to the GnRH test, pulsatile administration of GnRH can be used as a therapeutic modality. The presently proposed classification is presented graphically in Figure 3-1. It is our hope that it will serve the purpose for which it has been designed, i.e. to enable the proper classification of different types of anovulation using relatively simple and non-invasive methods and, consequently, the choice of the proper treatment from the available therapeutic armamentarium. In the discussion of various treatment

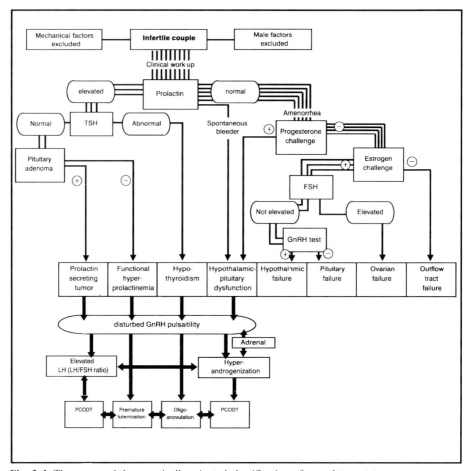

Fig. 3-1. The proposed therapeutically oriented classification of anovulatory states.

modalities used for the management of anovulatory states, in vitro fertilization (IVF) and other assisted reproduction techniques have not been included. The question of IVF as the ultimate modality in the treatment of infertility due to anovulation must, however, also be addressed. This method has been applied in recent years at many centers when other treatment protocols have failed to result in conception. Although its efficacy has been demonstrated, its logic seems still to be equivocal. It should yet be proven by well-controlled studies that, in cases of anovulatory infertility, IVF with its additional complications due to extracorporeal fertilization of the ovum is truly more efficient than properly planned and meticulously monitored ovulation induction therapy.

Elevated TSH may indicate the presence of subclinical hypothyroidism in hyperprolactinemic patients. Thyroid substitution therapy normalizes the prolactin levels and restores ovulatory cycles. Therefore this group has been included in the present classification system.

The basic experiments of Knobil (1980) demonstrated that proper pulsatile secretion of GnRH is essential for adequate pituitary and ovarian function. Any abnormality in GnRH pulsatility may lead to disturbances of gonadotropin secretion or follicular response and, consequently, may interfere with the sequence of events leading to ovulation. This leads to a whole array of interrelated pathologies which were previously classified as Hypothalamic-Pituitary Dysfunction (Group II). It has also been shown that a continuous hyperestrogenic environment, whatever its origin, will cause the pituitary to secrete LH in excess of FSH. This new knowledge made it necessary to subdivide the previously rather vaguely defined and multifactorial Group II (Hypothalamic-Pituitary Dysfunction).

Disturbed GnRH pulsatility in non-androgenized normoprolactinemic women is a common cause of ovulatory dysfunction (Oligo-anovulation). Treatment with clomiphene citrate is very effective in this subgroup. The effect of disturbed GnRH pulsatility depends also on the hormonal milieu of the pituitary gland and the sensitivity of different ovarian structures to gonadotropin stimulation. Incorporating this knowledge into the classification made it necessary to introduce 2 additional subgroups.

A specific category of anovulation is *premature luteinization*. This condition is frequently unrecognized or misdiagnosed as unexplained infertility, luteal phase defect, or luteinized unruptured follicle (LUF) syndrome. This situation will occur if an untimely LH surge appears in response to rising estrogen at a time when a follicle is still immature. It can only be diagnosed if an LH peak can be detected in the presence of an immature follicle, as seen on ultrasonography. Since stimulation by either clomiphene citrate or hMG cause multifollicular development with an exaggerated estrogen response, a premature LH peak is even more likely to occur during these stimulation regimens. This explains the relatively low success rate of clomiphene and hMG therapy in this subgroup of Hypothalamic-Pituitary Dysfunction. At present, this subgroup can be effectively treated with combined GnRH analog/gonadotropin therapy (see Chapters 4 and 7).

Disturbed GnRH pulsatility concomitant with excessive LH secretion may lead to *ovulation disturbances associated with hyper-androgenization.* It is also imaginable that this chain of events occurs in a reversed sequence.

The androgenized patient usually exhibits a past or present history of acne, seborrhea, and hirsutism which may or may not be associated with obesity. Investigation must be oriented towards identification of the source of the excessive androgens.

In patients with excessive androgens originating in the adrenals, as indicated by elevated dehydro-epiandrosterone-sulfate (DHEA-S), corticosteroids therapy will usually decrease androgens and, in consequence, normalize GnRH pulsatility and pituitary responsiveness and restore ovulation.

In androgenized women with normal or elevated total testosterone levels, elevated free testosterone, and normal DHEA-S levels, polycystic ovaries can be suspected. Sonographic imaging of the ovaries, preferably using the vaginal probe, permits a confirmation of this diagnosis. An elevated LH/FSH ratio (usually > 3) is also a characteristic feature of this diagnostic condition. The chronic elevated LH secretion may be initiated by increased androstendione/testosterone production or by peripheric conversion of androgens to estrone/estradiol (mainly in adipose tissue). However, a primary hypothalamic disorder should also be considered as an originator of the LH excess leading finally to PCOD.

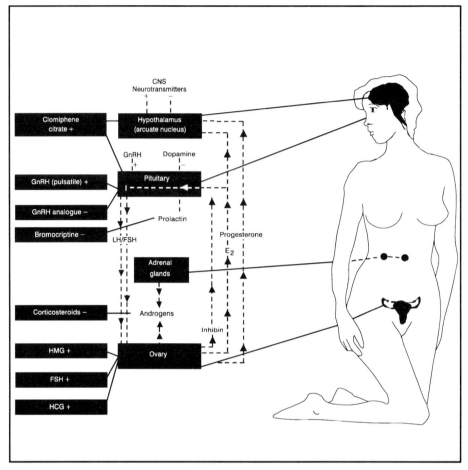

Fig. 3-2. Regulation of the female reproductive system and drugs used in the treatment of anovulation. The main target organs for the therapeutic agents are shown. (From: E. Lunenfeld and B. Lunenfeld, Modern approaches to the diagnosis and management of anovulation, Int. J. Fertil., 33:312, 1988.)

The first line therapy of PCOD, regardless of its etiology, is still clomiphene citrate (see Chapter 5). Despite an even further increase of LH activity, clomiphene will in some women allow the selection, growth, and maturation of a follicle. In some cases it will cause many follicles to develop and will result in hyperstimulation. In cases with inappropriate response to clomiphene citrate, gonadotropin therapy (preferably purified FSH) should be used in an attempt to override the FSH/LH imbalance. This therapy has a fair chance of success, although the incidence of hyperstimulation is increased (see Chapter 7). A more rational approach to the treatment of PCOD seems to be the induction of ovulation with gonadotropins following a long-term suppression of the pituitary-ovarian axis by potent GnRH analogs (see Chapters 4 and 7). It is, however, still not evident that even long-term pituitary suppression is capable of correcting the ovarian disease.

The inclusion of this specific subgroup of women with hypothalamic-pituitary-ovarian dysfunction within a framework of the classification will help in comparing the results obtained by different treatment modalities and protocols.

The above classification permits logical and efficient application of the presently available therapeutic armamentarium. Figure 3-2 shows the physiological mechanism of action of different ovulation-inducing agents as applied on the basis of the newly-proposed classification system.

4. GONADOTROPHIN-RELEASING HORMONE AND ITS ANALOGS

INTRODUCTION

Information arising in the central nervous system (CNS) or traveling through the bloodstream from other parts of the body culminates at the hypothalamus. The overall summation of these stimulatory and inhibiting signals results in the secretion of specific peptides from highly specialized hypothalamic neurons. These secretions, the releasing hormones, then stream along the neuron axon and are released at the nerve terminals located in the median eminence. There they are collected by the venous portal system and travel along the pituitary stalk to the anterior pituitary gland, where they exert their action.

In 1971, Schally's and Guillemin's groups reported the isolation, amino acid content, and later the sequence of luteinizing-releasing factor (LRF) (Burgus et al. 1971; Guillemin, 1978; Matsuo et al. 1971a; 1971b; Schally et al. 1978).

It is still not clear whether the hypothalamus secretes only one peptide capable of inducing the release of both LH and FSH or if there are two different releasing hormones, each for one gonadotrophin. The belief in one releasing hormone is widely accepted because administration of the highly purified native hormone or its synthetic analogs causes the secretion of both luteinizing hormone (LH) and follicle stimulating hormone (FSH) in vivo and in vitro (Herbert, 1976; Kao et al. 1977; Schally et al. 1971a; 1971b; 1971c).

BIOCHEMISTRY AND METABOLISM

GnRH is a decapeptide. Its amino acids sequence is shown in Figure 4-1. The spatial structure of the molecule and its receptor-binding characteristics are determined by the pyroglutamic acid in position 1 and by the amino acids in positions 4 to 10. The histidine and tryptophan acids in positions 2 and 3 are crucial in determining the molecular activity and substitution of these two amino acids results in numerous analogs that differ from the natural molecule by higher or lower activity.

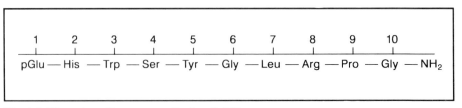

Fig. 4-1. The aminoacids sequence of native GnRH.

A simple D-amino acid substitution in position 6 is common to most agonists. Many are nine amino acid peptides, the glycine in position 10 being replaced by an ethylamide group. These simple modifications impart an increase in binding affinity to pituitary GnRH receptors and/or an increased resistance to the proteolytic degradation that rapidly destroys native GnRH. Substitution of several amino acids or changing the GnRH by reducing the size of the amino acid chain may produce materials with biological action opposite to that of the native hormone (GnRH antagonists). Up till now, more than 2000 GnRH analogs have been produced and more than a dozen are commercially available (Fig. 4-2).

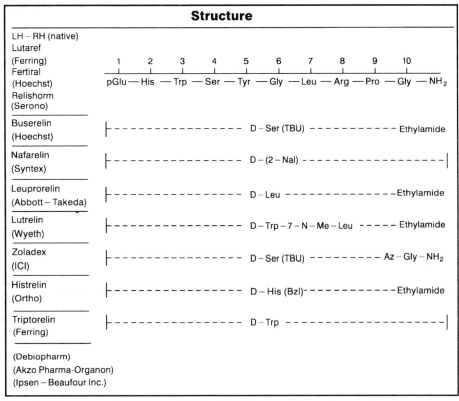

Fig. 4-2. The aminoacids sequence of native GnRH compared to analogs produced at present by various pharmaceutical companies.

GnRH is transported by the venous portal system to the pituitary where it exerts its action and is then degraded.

Although the GnRH molecule appears to be designed for a rather long biologic half-life, because of the pyroglutamic residue blocking the amino end of the molecule to protect it from degradation by aminopeptidases and because of the amide function to protect the carboxyl end of the peptide from degradation by carboxypeptidases, native GnRH has a very short half-life. This is due to the fact that brain enzymes inactivate GnRH at the Gly6 Leu7 bond very rapidly (Hazum et al. 1981; Koch et al. 1974).

GnRH is also metabolized in the kidney, as shown by in vivo studies with tritiated GnRH (Redding et al. 1973) and by the observation that the clearance rate of exogenous GnRH was calculated to be $1{,}640 \pm 60$ ml/min. and the plasma half-life to be 5.5 to 8.0 minutes in the normal subject (Pimstone et al. 1977).

The portal vein concentration of GnRH in the rhesus monkey was measured by Carmel and colleagues (1976). During the early follicular phase, they found basal levels of 66.0 ± 6.6 pg/ml interrupted by rapid rises in concentration (pulses) of up to 200 pg/ml. In patients undergoing transsphenoidal surgery, they found levels ranging from undetectable to 1000 pg/ml.

CELLULAR MECHANISM OF ACTION

The gonadotrophs comprise 10 to 15 % of the total number of pituitary cells, and GnRH binds selectively to these cells (Naor et al. 1982).

The initial response of the gonadotroph to a GnRH stimulus is brisk and when the signal fades, the cell stops releasing the hormone. This short stimulation is possible because of the rapid degradation of GnRH at the pituitary level.

The main stages of GnRH action upon the gonadotrophins are schematically presented in Figure 4-3. The decapeptide binds to specific receptors situated in the cell membrane. The hormone-receptor complex is then internalized into the cell. It seems that a specific G-1 protein enhances this process by coupling with the HR complex. Following the internalization of GnRH into the gonadotroph, the first

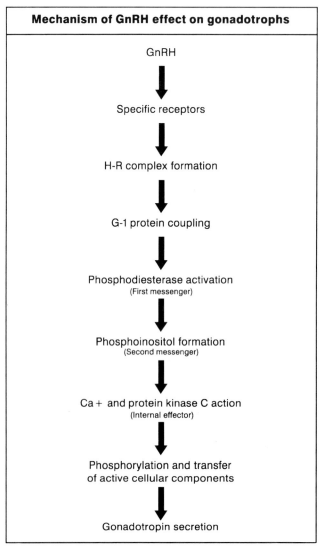

Fig. 4–3. Mechanism of GnRH effect on gonadotrophins

messenger of hormonal effect, i.e. phosphodiesterase, is activated, and phosphoinositol (second messenger) is formed. The next step is dependent on the action of the protein kinase C (internal effector).

This step also requires the presence of active calcium ions, which on the one hand are mobilized from the intracellular reservoir and, on the other hand, are supplied from outside the cell. The latter function is made possible by the opening and activation of special channels in the cell membrane. Specific cell components are now phosphorylated and transferred into the required position (Naor et al. 1989). The effect of all the above changes is the mobilization and transfer of FSH- and LH-containing granules through the cell membrane and, consequently, the secretion of these hormones into the blood stream.

GnRH has been shown not only to induce the secretion of gonadotrophins but also to participate in their synthesis. Liu and Jackson (1978) showed that, in the rat, GnRH had an impact on the incorporation of carbohydrate residues (mainly sialic acid) into the molecule. They demonstrated that the carbohydrate content of LH released in response to GnRH stimulation differed from that released in the absence of exogenous GnRH and that there were two pools of secretable LH: stored and newly-synthesized. The two could be differentiated by the carbohydrate content of their molecules. The newly synthesized releasable molecule contained more carbohydrate than the stored one and was biologically more active.

PATTERN OF GnRH SECRETION

GnRH is secreted from the hypothalamus in a pulsatile fashion (i.e., short periods of abrupt secretion separated by longer periods of low or undetectable secretion). The plasma levels of immunoreactive endogenous LHRH in women were measured by Elkind-Hirsch and colleagues (1982) and found to be cyclic with a frequency approximating one pulse per hour.

The frequency and amplitude of the GnRH pulse are crucial for the release of LH and FSH. Knobil's group (Pohl et al. 1983) demonstrated that intermittent administration of exogenous GnRH to monkeys with arcuate nucleus lesions reestablished the gonadotropin pulsatile secretion and the peripheral plasma level. Continuous administration of the releasing-hormone at various infusion rates failed to restore gonadotropin secretion. Furthermore, in ovariectomized hypothalamic lesioned monkeys, changing the GnRH pulse frequency itself or its amplitude had a direct influence on the secretion and relative amount of each of the gonadotropins. Thus, raising the frequency from the physiologic one pulse per hour rate to three or five pulses per hour reduced the secretion of both LH and FSH. Lowering the frequency to one pulse every 3 hours caused a variable decline in LH levels but not in FSH levels, which, in fact, rose. Lowering the exogenous GnRH pulse amplitude while keeping the pulse frequency at the physiologic rate resulted in a decline of both gonadotropins to undetectable levels. Raising the pulse amplitude under these conditions lowered the FSH levels but not the LH levels (Wildt et al. 1981). It seems from this experimental model that the fashion in which the pituitary is challenged by GnRH determines its secretory reaction.

DIAGNOSTIC USE OF GnRH

GnRH acts directly on the pituitary and, when administered intravenously as a bolus, tests the size of the releasable pool of pituitary gonadotrophin (Figs. 4-4 and 4-5). It is

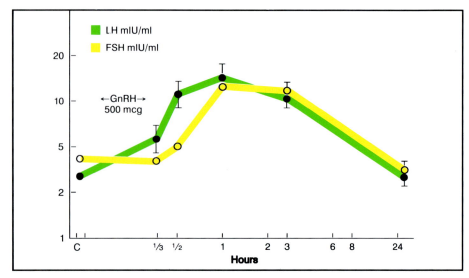

Fig. 4-4. Positive response to GnRH administration in a patient with primary amenorrhea. This patient belonged to Group I. She had low endogenous estrogen and gonadotropins, did not respond to the administration of clomiphene citrate and had no withdrawal bleeding after administration of medroxy-progesterone-acetate (MAP). A positive response to GnRH indicated that the main lesion was not at the pituitary level. As expected, she did respond to direct stimulation of ovaries with hMG/hCG and conceived when so treated. (C = Control levels)

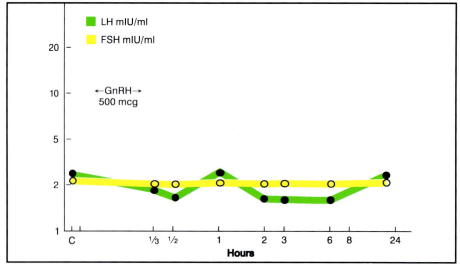

Fig. 4-5. Negative response to single GnRH administration in a patient with primary amenorrhea. This patient belonged to Group I. She had low endogenous estrogen and gonadotropins, did not respond to the administration of clomiphene citrate and had no withdrawal bleeding after administration of medroxy-progesterone-acetate (MAP). Lack of response to GnRH indicated that the main lesion could be located in the pituitary. As expected, she did respond to direct stimulation of the ovaries with hMG/hCG and conceived when so treated. (C = Control levels)

important to recognize that when the pituitary has not been previously primed by GnRH, this response to GnRH may not occur. Where there is no response, one has to rule out the possibility of depletion of pituitary gonadotrophin content. In such cases, continued stimulation with GnRH is called for prior to performing the standard GnRH test.

The standard test for adults is to administer 100 mg of GnRH intravenously in a bolus and then to obtain blood samples for gonadotrophin assays every 15 minutes for 1 hour. In adult females, the response observed varies with the phase of the menstrual cycle. In the early follicular phase, a three- to four-fold increase is observed in serum LH, while in the preovulatory period the increments can be much higher. Since LH-release is modulated by estrogens, one might suspect that this difference in response is due to higher estrogen levels normally found in the latter part of the follicular phase. The test has some value in the localization of lesions in the hypothalamic-hypophyseal axis. However, it seems that the initial high hopes for the diagnostic value of GnRH in amenorrheic patients have not been fulfilled. Consensus has now been reached that amenorrheic women do not require a dynamic test with GnRH unless one is planning to induce ovulation by chronic intermittent infusion of this hormone.

THERAPEUTIC APPLICATIONS IN WOMEN

The use of GnRH can be considered for patients lacking endogenous gonadotropins who have a pituitary gland capable of responding to this medication. Thus, GnRH has a place in the treatment of hypothalamic amenorrhea.

In 1971, Kastin et al. reported the use of GnRH to evoke sufficient LH secretion to induce ovulation in an amenorrheic patient after follicular growth and maturation was stimulated by hMG. The patient conceived and delivered a healthy baby. Since then, a number of similarly induced ovulations and pregnancies have terminated in the births of healthy babies. It should be noted that all the women in this group exhibited endogenous estrogen activity before the commencement of the treatment. Administration of GnRH alone has been used for the treatment of infertility in hypothalamic amenorrhea and anorexia nervosa (Nillius & Wide, 1979); however, its effectiveness has been limited.

The search of the early literature regarding the clinical use of nonpulsatile GnRH therapy revealed that in 218 trials only 67 ovulations and 14 conceptions occurred.

Thus, the initial high hopes for GnRH therapy were not fulfilled, and the general interest in this approach to treatment declined. Lack of the expected clinical responses to nonpulsatile administration of GnRH, even in high doses, is not surprising in view of the concept of down regulation. Early experiments with GnRH agonist showed that initial stimulation of gonadotrophin release was followed by return to baseline levels or below. Receptor-binding studies showed that the latter effect was due to a decrease in the number of receptors on the cell and not to an alteration of the affinity of receptors for GnRH (Belchetz et al. 1978). This phenomenon has been exploited by using potent GnRH-agonists to induce a gonadotrophin-specific temporary hypophysectomy (Crowley et al. 1980; Borgman et al. 1982; Shadmi et al. 1987; Insler et al. 1988).

Following Knobil's (1980) demonstration that imitation of the physiologic pulsatile pattern of GnRH could restore ovarian function in the hypothalamus-lesioned monkeys, interest in the therapeutic use of GnRH was again stimulated.

TABLE 4-1. Results obtained with intermittent GnRH at different Dosages and Treatment Schedules

Author	No. of patients	Dosage/pulse (μg)	Interval (min)	Pulses (24 hrs)	Route*)	No. of cycles	No. of ovulations	No. of pregnancies
Crowley and McArthur (1980)	3	1.5-3	120	12	SC	3	3	–
Leyendecker et al. (1980)	8	2.5-5-10-15-20	89	16	IV	26	26	6
Keogh et al. (1981)	1	3.4	62.5	23	SC	1	1	1
Nillius et al. (1981)	14	500	480	3	SC	14	11	2
Schoemaker et al. (1982)	9	100	120	9	IV	8	5	–
Schoemaker et al. (1982)	9	20	120	9	IV	20	17	5
Schoemaker et al. (1982)	9	20	96	15	IV	3	3	1
Schoemaker et al. (1982)	9	10	90	16	IV	1	1	–
Skarin et al. (1982)	6	20	90	16	SC	16	7	1
Berg et al. (1983)	27	20	90	16	IV	40	32	11
Weber et al. (1983)	5	10-20	90	16	IV	5	4	–
Coelingh-Bennink (1983)	11	10-40	90	16	IV	27	19	7
Miller et al. (1983)	8	1-5	96-120	12-16	IV	23	20	5
Blankstein et al. (1986)	295	12.5-25.0	90	16	IV	516	405	135

*) SC = subcutaneous; IV = intravenous.

Leyendecker et al. (1980; 1980b) showed that it was possible to induce ovulation followed by pregnancy in an amenorrheic patient with hypothalamic failure by pulsatile intravenous administration of GnRH through a computerized infusion pump. During the last few years a number of reports on the pulsatile administration of GnRH have appeared (Table 4-1).

Technique

GnRH is administered by a computerized portable minipump attached to an indwelling intravenous or subcutaneous catheter. Frequent monitoring of the patient is necessary in order to detect whether there are any complications from the pump (phlebitis, local inflammation, etc.) and to ensure that the pump functions well. The pulse frequency and dose are adjusted to the patient's response. Dosages and pulse frequencies used by various authors are shown in Table 4-1. Periodic measurement of serum FSH and LH can show whether the pituitary responds normally and adequately to the pulsatile GnRH stimulation. The response to pulsatile administration of GnRH is reflected by the elevation of serum FSH and LH secretion and by an anatomic growth of follicles accompanied by biochemical changes mainly with respect to increased synthesis and secretion of steroid hormones. The follicular enlargement can be visualized by ultrasonographic measurements, and estrogen secretions can be estimated directly by their measurement in urine or blood, or indirectly by their effect on secondary targets such as the cervical mucus.

The patient is instructed to record basal temperature daily. This will permit detection of the day of presumed ovulation, allow an assessment of the length of the luteal phase, and help determine the day when blood should be drawn for progesterone (day 5-8 post nadir). It will also indicate whether a pregnancy can be suspected and when hCG determination should be performed, as well as establish when treatment should be stopped. Cervical score (Insler et al. 1972) should be estimated periodically from the fifth day on, in order to detect the initial estrogenic activity. This will assist in recognizing when the active phase of follicular growth started. When the cervical score is above 8 points, monitoring is continued by estrogen determination. When urinary estrogen levels reach about 80 μg/24 hrs., or when serum estradiol is 250 pg/ml, ultrasonographic visualization of the ovaries should be undertaken. All these measurements make it possible to assess the time of ovulation and to decide on the optimal timing of coitus. At this point the patient is instructed to have sexual intercourse and to return to the clinic between 2 and 10 hours thereafter. During the visit a cervical mucus sample is taken, the cervical score estimated, and a postcoital test performed. Treatment with GnRH may be interrupted whenever a satisfactory follicular diameter is reached and estrogen levels are in an acceptable range, at which time hCG is administered. Another possibility is to suspend GnRH administration after ovulation has occurred. hCG is then applied in order to support the developing corpus luteum (Leyendecker et al. 1980).

Results

The results obtained by treatment with chronic intermittent (pulsatile) GnRH administration are summarized in Table 4-1.

Nillius et al. (1981) treated 14 amenorrheic women with no signs of endogenous estrogen production by giving chronic intermittent therapy with 500 mg of GnRH subcutaneously at 8 hour pulses for 28 days. Follicle maturation and ovulation were induced in 11 women, 2 of whom became pregnant during the course of treatment. Leyendecker et al. (1980) treated 8 women, 4 of whom were suffering from primary and 4 from secondary hypothalamic amenorrhea. The patients were treated by chronic intermittent, intravenous administration of GnRH with doses of 2.5, 5, 10, 15, or 20 μg of GnRH every 90 minutes over a period of 6 to 16 days. The dose was adjusted to each patient individually by monitoring the pituitary and ovarian response. This study demonstrated that different patients may require different amounts of GnRH, although the pulse frequency was equal in all patients. Patients who, prior to treatment, exhibited a significant response to a 100 μg test dose of GnRH seemed to respond well to doses of 10 to 15 μg of GnRH per pulse. The duration of chronic intermittent treatment required for induction of ovulation in these patients was 6 to 8 days. With this regimen, ovulation was obtained in all 26 treatment cycles, and out of the 8 women treated, 6 conceived. Crowley & McArthur (1980) treated 3 patients with Kallman's syndrome with subcutaneous bihourly pulses of 25 to 50 μg per kilogram of GnRH. They succeeded in inducing ovulation in all three cycles.

Skarin et al. (1982) treated a group of 6 normoprolactinemic women with secondary amenorrhea of 2 1/2 to 11 years' duration, all lacking endogenous gonadotropin. The patients received 20 μg of GnRH every 20 minutes through a chronic indwelling catheter inserted subcutaneously in the fat tissue of the abdominal wall. The therapy was continued until menstruation occurred or pregnancy was ascertained. All women responded to the pulsatile GnRH therapy with follicular maturation. Ovulation occurred following 8 to 23 days' treatment (median 14 days), and one patient conceived. One patient developed hyperstimulation during her first treatment cycle. Schoemaker et al. (1982) reported on different doses and different pulse intervals in 32 treatment cycles. By administering 100 μg of GnRH every 120 minutes, they achieved five ovulations in eight cycles, but no pregnancies. With this treatment regimen, the authors found that the LH response showed a preovulatory dip and that both LH and FSH peaks were lower than those observed when 20 μg of GnRH were administered every 120 minutes. With the latter treatment regimen they achieved 17 ovulations in 20 cycles, and five pregnancies occurred. With 20 μg of GnRH intravenously every 96 minutes they achieved three ovulations and one pregnancy in three cycles. With 10 μg of GnRH intravenously each 20 minutes, one ovulation occurred, but no pregnancy resulted. Reviewing 36 papers published between 1980 and 1984 (Blankstein et al. 1986), 916 treatment cycles in 388 patients could be assessed. The conception rate was 56 %, multiple gestation rate 7.3 %, abortion rate 14.5 %, and hyperstimulation rate 1.1 %. Although it appears that careful monitoring will reduce the appearance of hyperstimulation, more cases have to be evaluated before definite conclusions can be drawn. From reviews of the available literature, it seems that doses between 5.0 and 20.0 μg, with pulse intervals between 62.5 and 120.0 minutes, are capable of eliciting pituitary response sufficient for follicular stimulation resulting in ovulation.

Side Effects

Although the number of treatment cycles reported is still small, the review of the literature enables one to point out a number of possible complications: (1) Occasional phlebitis (rarely accompanied by bacteremia) may occur in cases in which the catheter was inserted intravenously, (2) ovarian cysts developed in a few patients, (3) cases of hyperstimulation were reported, and (4) failure due to mechanical defects was noted. Specifically, there were temporary interruptions of the pump function that resulted in periodic discontinuation of GnRH, causing luteal deficiencies expressed clinically by short luteal phases. Thus, in order to obtain optimal results with chronic intermittent administration of GnRH, careful monitoring of pituitary and ovarian responses is necessary.

GnRH ANALOGS: AGONISTS AND ANTAGONISTS

The main reason for the tremendous amount of interest in GnRH and its analogs during the past decade is the fact that, depending on their mode of application, they can either stimulate pituitary gonadotrophin secretion or be potent inhibitors. When administered in a precise pulsatile pattern, GnRH can restore the normal cyclic gonadotrophin secretion. When administered chronically, GnRH or its agonists proved to be potent inhibitors of gonadotrophin secretion, providing a gonadotrophin-specific, temporary (fully reversible) medical hypophysectomy (Cetel et al. 1983; Karten & Rivier, 1986) The possibility of achieving a temporary medical hypophysectomy has been used as a rationale for consequently attaining a medical gonadectomy, i.e. for temporarily shutting off the gonadal steroids production. This could be of value in the treatment of diseases dependent on gonadal steroids. To date, indeed, this approach has proven its efficacy in the treatment of metastatic prostatic cancer (Soloway et al. 1988), precocious puberty (Laron et al. 1988; Aubert et al. 1988), and endometriosis (Dmowski et al. 1988; Brosens & Cornillie, 1988). It has been shown to reduce the volume of uterine fibroids (leiomyomata) and has been suggested as a medical therapy for this condition in high risk surgical cases of perimenopausal women (Healy, 1986). It is being investigated for hormone-dependent breast cancer (Klijn et al. 1988; Robertson & Blamey, 1988) and for ovarian cancer (Emons, 1988; Jaeger, 1988).

In the management of the infertile patient, where conventional treatment regimes had failed, GnRH agonists have been successfully utilized to suppress the pituitary ovarian axis, prior to and concomitantly with stimulation of follicular growth and induction of ovulation by exogenous gonadotropins (see Chapter 7).

This therapeutic regime has also been efficiently used for the stimulation of multiple follicular development in in vitro fertilization programs, to prevent dropouts due to an untimely LH surge (Insler et al. 1988; Lunenfeld et al. 1988).

GnRH agonists have been dispersed in biocompatible biodegradable polymeric matrixes of DL-lactide-coglycolide in the form of microcapsules or microspheres. Alternatively, they are incorporated in a matrix of lactide-glycolide co-polymers in the form of biodegradable implants. The introduction of potent and long-acting agonists and delayed release formulations has permitted application on a once-per-month basis for long-term treatment of gonadal steroids-dependent diseases described above (Parmar et al. 1988; Max et al. 1988; Friedman et al. 1988). This has improved their usefulness and acceptance.

While the availability of potent GnRH agonists has resulted in their widespread clinical use during the last few years, the production of suitable antagonists working by receptor occupancy has been disappointing. Progress in the synthesis of antagonists was slower, since several amino acids have to be substituted on the GnRH molecule. Antagonists also require precise topological features for high binding affinity to the receptor. GnRH antagonists with their immediate inhibitory actions may be useful for contraception and in treatment of hormone-dependent disorders as described above, avoiding the initial stimulatory phase of the agonist.

The present disadvantage of antagonists is that their effective dosage is approximately 1000 times that of agonists. Furthermore, introducing of DArg or other basic side chains into position 6 induced cutaneous anaphylactoid-like reactions and has been shown to trigger histamine release from rat mast cells. Recently, attempts have been made to synthesize GnRH antagonists lacking the histamine-releasing activity. This was achieved by either switching the residues between positions 5 and 6 or by reducing the overall hydrophobicity and shielding the side chain basic groups.

TABLE 4-2. GnRH Antagonists, lacking histamine-releasing activity, available in 1992 for clinical trias.

GnRH native	pGlu 1	His 2	Trp 3	Ser 4	Tyr 5	Gly 6	Leu 7	Arg 8	Pro 9	GlyNH2 10
GnRH antagonistes:										
Nal–Glu (Ortho)	NAcD2Nal	DpClPhe	D3Pal	●	Arg	D-Gly	●	●	●	D-Ala
Nal–Lys (Serono)	NAcD2Nal	DpClPhe	D3Pal	●	NicLys	D-NicLys	●	ILys	●	D-Ala
ORG 30850 (Organon)	AcDCpa	Dcpa	DBta	●	●	D-Lys	●	●	●	D-Ala
SB 075 (Schally)	NAcD2Nal	DpClPhe	D3Pal	●	●	D-Cit	●	●	●	D-Ala
RS 26306 (Syntex)	NAcD2Nal	DpClPhe	D3Pal	●	●	D-hArg (Et2)	●	L-hArg (Et2)	●	D-Ala
MGE 013 (Hoechst)	NAcD2Nal	DpClPhe	D-Trp	●	●	D-Ser (RHA)	●	●	●	AzGly

With all the tremendous potential of GnRH analogs in the treatment of a wide variety of sex steroid-dependent disorders, prolonged decrease of estrogen may lead to deleterious metabolic disturbances. Changes in lipid metabolism and decrease in bone mineral content have been observed with prolonged use. The development of adjunctive treatment regimes may be necessary to prevent these effects. If long-acting formulations become available and long-term safety can be assured, GnRH agonists and antagonists could also provide an effective alternative in male and female contraception.

Well-controlled long-term postmarketing surveillance will be necessary to demonstrate that GnRH analog therapy is safe. If so proven, these agents can provide a revolutionary approach to sex hormone-dependent diseases and a manifold impact on present therapy.

5. COMPOUNDS WITH ESTROGEN-LIKE ACTIVITY

EPIMESTROL

Epimestrol (EL) is a synthetic derivative of the naturally-occurring estrogen, estriol. Its proper chemical name is 3-Methoxy-17-epiestriol (Fig. 5-1). When administered in a dose of 5 to 20 mg daily for a number of days following spontaneous or induced bleeding, this compound may induce ovulation in some anovulatory women.

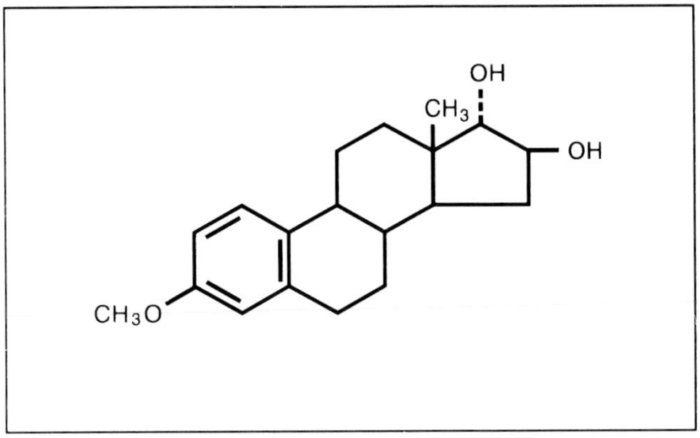

Fig. 5-1. Chemical structure of 3-Methoxy-17-Epiestriol (Epimestrol®).

   The mechanism of epimestrol's action upon the hypothalamic-pituitary-ovarian axis and its effect on the genital tract are still not established in sufficient detail. Darmasetiawan et al. (1985) suggested that the compound acts at the receptor levels increasing the number of receptors and improving the process of steroidogenesis. Kloosterboer et al. (1985) examined the influence of various doses of epimestrol on estrogen and progesterone receptors in ovariectomized rats pretreated with estradiol. They found that a low dose of EL increased both estrogen and progesterone receptors and that uterine weight was significantly increased one day following application of the drug.
   D'Ambrogio et al. (1987) found that, particularly in PCOD patients, epimestrol modulated the frequency of LH pulses to a range between 50 and 135 min, reduced the overall LH levels, and improved the FSH/LH ratio. Genazzani & D'Ambrogio (1986) reported that, in girls with delayed puberty, administration of 1.25–2.5 mg b.i.d of EL for several weeks induced a progressive increase of gonadotropin levels. Nappi et al. (1981) and our own experience (Insler et al. 1973) showed that epimestrol had no adverse effects on cervical mucus production. Nitschke-Dabelstein et al. (1981) indicated that treatment of anovulation using epimestrol resulted in monofollicular development without the occurrence of multifollicular cycles. According to our knowledge, there were no reports of ovarian hyperstimulation or other serious side effects following epimestrol treatment.
   Various authors report that the efficacy of epimestrol in inducing ovulation and/or conception in infertile patients seems to vary greatly (Table 5-1). The ovulation rates range from 30 to 100% and pregnancy rates from 0 to 61% (median 20%). The

TABLE 5–1. Results of Treatment with Epimestrol in various Types of Ovulation Disturbances (% or absolute numbers)

Authors (Year)	No. of Patients	Type of Disturbance	Ovulations	Conceptions
Gimes & Toth (1973)	37	Anovulation	96 %	16
Insler et al. (1973)	23	Anovulation	41 %	0
Keller (1975a)	53	WHO Group II	30 %	?
Koehler (1980)	49	Infertility	42	30
Cortes-Prieto et al. (1981)	10	Anovulation	?	2
Lopes et al. (1981)	21	WHO Group II	49 %	4
Hammerstein & Schmidt (1981)	653	Anovulation C. L. defic.		126
Bohnet et al. (1981)	17	C. L. defic.	10	2
Aksu (1982)	21	Anovulation	15	9
Maia et al. (1983)	10	Anovulation	6	5
Darmasetiawan et al. (1985)	24	Anovulation Oligomenor. Amenorrhea	100 % 54 % 0	? ? 0
Graf et al. (1986)	11	Amenorrhea	0	0
Zrubek et al. (1986)	73	WHO Group II	38	14
Ambrogio et al. (1987)	18	PCO	83 %	?

existing bias is also augmented by the use of EL in combination with hCG (Lopez et al. 1981), clomiphene (Bullietti et al. 1986), single doses of GnRH (Maia et al. 1983) and bromocriptine (Polatti, 1981). Most of the authors, however, agree that EL is not capable of inducing ovulation in amenorrheic women with hypothalamic-pituitary failure (WHO Group I) (Graf et al. 1986; Darmasetiawan et al. 1985).

It seems that the mechanism of action of epimestrol has not yet been studied in sufficient detail. The selection of patients, treatment regimes, and monitoring methods have not yet been clarified. For the above reasons, it seems justified to conclude that epimestrol may be used as a cycle regulator in patients complaining of menstrual disorders (excluding amenorrhea). However, when the primary complaint is infertility, more efficient ovulation inducers should be applied.

CYCLOFENIL

Cyclofenil (Bis-(p-Acetoxyfenyl)-Cyclohexylidenmethan) is structurally related to the potent synthetic estrogen diethylstilbestrol (Fig. 5-2). It was shown to induce FSH-release in rats (Yaoi and Bettendorf, 1973) and cause an increase of gonadotrophin levels in the human (Person, 1965; Neale et al. 1970). Cyclofenil is a weak estrogen and, unlike clomiphene citrate, has no antiestrogenic properties. This lack of antiestrogenic properties is evidenced by the secretion of copious, thin, elastic cervical mucus observed during treatment with cyclofenil (Sato et al. 1969). The drug is administered in a dosage of 400–600 mg daily for periods of 5 to 10 days every month, or 200 mg given continuously for several months.

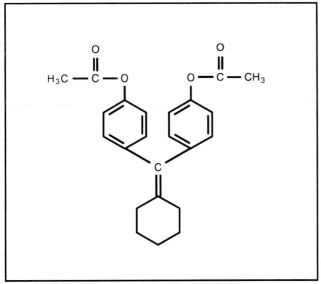

Fig. 5–2. Chemical structure of Bis-(p-Acetoxyphenyl)-Cyclohexylidenmethan (Cyclofenil).

As far as ovulation induction is concerned, cyclofenil seems to be fairly effective. Ploman (1973) reported an ovulation rate of 57.3% and a pregnancy rate of 26.7% in a group of 75 patients treated over 434 cycles during 4 years. Berger (1972) claimed the ovulation rate to be 75%; exceptionally high in comparison to other reports. Neale et al. (1970) observed biphasic cycles in 31% of treated patients. Schmidt-Elmendorff (1971) reported an ovulation rate of 64% and a pregnancy rate of 32%. Sato et al. (1969) reported an ovulation rate of 43% and a pregnancy rate of 14%. The drug seems to cause only a few side effects. Hyperstimulation syndrome was not observed. Less than 1% of patients complained of nausea, hot flashes, or slight abdominal pain (Keller, 1975a, 1975b). Some cases of mild cholestatic jaundice, possibly connected with cyclofenil treatment, were reported (Ploman, 1973). Such symptoms regressed rapidly in all cases following cessation of therapy.

Like epimestrol, cyclofenil may be used for the amelioration of mild cycle disturbances. However, there is no doubt that for induction of ovulation in patients belonging to Group II, the treatment of choice is still clomiphene citrate.

CLOMIPHENE CITRATE AND RELATED DRUGS

Historical Background

In 1937, Robson and Schonberg (1937) reported in *Nature* that triphenylethylene and triphenylchloroethylene are estrogen agonists of low potency but of long duration of action. These observations received little attention until 1953, when Shelton et al. (1953) demonstrated that the biologic potency of the estrogen agonists could be augmented by alkoxy substitution. Six years later, Allen et al. (1959) obtained a patent for clomiphene citrate, a triphenylethylene derivative substituted with a chloride anion and an amino alkoxyl.

The first clinical trials of ovulation induction were carried out in 1961 with MER–25, a close structural analog of clomiphene, by Kistner and Smith (1961). It was in October of 1961 that Robert Greenblatt and his coworkers reported in the *Journal of the American Medical Association* the first results of clinical testing with clomiphene, which was then known as MRL–41. This was the first publication on the clinical action of this drug. Greenblatt reported that "although the mechanism of action of this compound is not clear at the present time, it is heartening to find a drug which holds much promise of inducing ovulatory type menses with considerable regularity in anovulatory women." Greenblatt et al. (1961) were the first to report the successful induction of ovulation and pregnancies following clomiphene therapy. Subsequently, other pharmacologic agents for ovulation induction were developed, but clomiphene citrate has probably helped more infertile women to conceive than any other mode of infertility therapy.

Chemistry and Pharmacology

Clomiphene citrate (CC) is a white or pale yellow, odorless powder whith a melting point of 116-118 °C. It has a molecular weight of 598.1 daltons and is unstable in air and light. Clomiphene is a triarylethylene compound (1-p-diethyl aminoethoxyphenyl- 1,2-diphenyl-2-chloroethylene citrate) chemically related to chlorotrianisene (TACE), which is a weak estrogen. Structurally, it is related to the potent synthetic estrogen diethylstilbestrol. Clomiphene may exist in either the (cis) zuclomiphene or the (trans) enclomiphene configuration, the former being significantly more potent. In the preparations commercially available, the isomers are in the ratio of 40% zu- and 60% enclomiphene (Fig. 5-3). It is not known how the various parts of the molecule contribute to clomiphene's action. It is known, however, that, while the EN(trans) isomer has antiestrogen and weakly estrogenic properties, the ZU(cis) isomer exerts only estrogenic effects. It is worth noting that, at recommended doses, clomiphene citrate does not display significant estrogenic activity in the human.

Tamoxifen p-(dimethylaminoethoxyphenyl- 1,2-diphenylbut-1 ene), is structurally related to clomiphene citrate and seems to act in a similar manner. It is a potent antiestrogen which has been widely used in the therapy of metastasizing and inoperable mammary cancer, since it inhibits the binding of estradiol to its receptor in mammary and uterine tissue (McGuire & De la Garcia, 1973).

Tracer studies of clomiphene with radioactive carbon labeling have shown that the main route of excretion is by the feces, although small amounts are also excreted in urine. There is strong evidence that clomiphene is concentrated in the bile and carried by it into the gut. Reabsorption takes place from the gut, so that clomiphene is to some extent sequestered in an enterohepatic circulation, from which it leaks out slowly. After intravenous administration, 37% is excreted in 5 days. The appearance of 14C in the feces 6 weeks after administration suggests that the remaining drug and/or metabolites are slowly excreted from a sequestered enterohepatic recirculation pool (Swyer, 1965).

Geier et al. (1987) have developed a radioreceptor assay suitable for measuring of antiestrogens such as clomiphene and tamoxiphene at the same time as their active metabolites in serum. Estrogens as well as antiestrogens show a relatively high binding affinity to estrogen receptors. The assay is based on the capability of antiestrogen to displace radio-labelled estradiol from an estrogen receptor preparation. The amount of antiestrogen is expressed as estradiol-binding equivalent, i.e. pgE2 displaced from the receptor.

Sequential blood samples were obtained from five volunteers with ovarian failure who received a single oral dose of 100 mg clomiphene citrate. Following the administration of clomiphene for 5 consecutive days at a dose of 100 mg daily, the drug could be detected in serum for up to 30 days.

At the time of ovulation and following nidation, elevated amounts of endogenous estrogens are present, hence it could be assumed that the amount of clomiphene present at that time will in most cases not be sufficient to displace enough estrogen to endanger the oocyte or estrogen-sensitive tissue during embryogenesis.

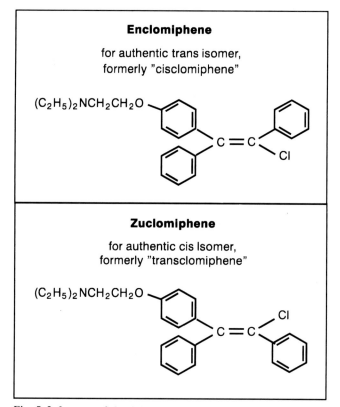

Enclomiphene

for authentic trans isomer,
formerly "cisclomiphene"

$(C_2H_5)_2NCH_2CH_2O$

Zuclomiphene

for authentic cis Isomer,
formerly "transclomiphene"

$(C_2H_5)_2NCH_2CH_2O$

Fig. 5–3. Isomers of clomiphene.

Following the development of a reverse phase high pressure liquid chromatography (HPLC) assay that could distinguish the CC isomers (Mickelson et al. 1984), a comparison of the pharmacokinetic disposition of the ZU and EN isomers of CC was performed (Mickelson et al. 1986). It is apparent that each isomer exhibits its own characteristic pharmacokinetic profile, the EN isomer being absorbed faster and eliminated more completely than the ZU isomer. Although CC tablets consist to 62% of the EN isomer and 38% of the ZU isomer, the observed plasma concentrations of the ZU isomer were much higher than those of the EN isomer. Because the ZU isomer is considered more estrogenic than the EN isomer, response of the target tissues should vary according to both the relative affinity and the concentrations of each isomer interacting with the relevant estrogen receptor.

Mode of Action

Cellular Effects

It is claimed that the main effect of clomiphene is competition with estrogen for binding sites on the acceptor molecules which bind the receptor to DNA.

The stereoscopic configuration of clomiphene citrate is sufficiently similar to that of estradiol to compete with it for available estrogen receptor sites in all estrogen-dependent target cells in the hypothalamus, pituitary, ovary, uterus, and cervical epithelium. Not only does clomiphene limit the availability of the receptors to estrogen, but the binding of clomiphene also shifts the equilibrium of the receptors from the nonactivated and activated states toward the nonactivated state (Sasson & Notides, 1982). Once clomiphene successfully binds to the estrogen acceptor molecules in the nucleus, it induces a subtle, though important conformational change in the receptor, which alters the receptor-complex's ability to associate with some chromatin components, thus affecting the normal events of expression. Since the receptor-clomiphene complex cannot form the requisite allosteric configuration, its nuclear interaction differs from that of estrogens and results only in limited estrogenic responses (Sutherland, 1981). Clomiphene cannot induce the synthesis of estrogen receptors, an effect which Katzenellenbogen et al. (1979) claim is the drug's most important antiestrogen property. Moreover, the clomiphene-receptor complex in the nucleus is associated with long-term inhibition of the normal recycling of receptors from the nucleus to the cytoplasm. Clomiphene thus causes estrogen-insensitivity in the target cells. The diminished ability of the cell to respond to estrogen is compounded by the fact that clomiphene, not being a natural estrogen, is unable to generate and transmit a meaningful estrogenic message to the nuclear apparatus of estrogen-dependent target cells.

Effects on the Hypothalamic-Pituitary-Ovarian Axis

The mode of action of clomiphene in the induction of ovulation may be tentatively described as follows. Blinded by clomiphene molecules occupying the estrogen receptor sites, the hypothalamus and pituitary are unable to correctly perceive the real level of estrogens in the blood. A false message of insufficient estrogen concentration is registered and acted upon, resulting in exaggerated secretion of FSH and LH. When clomiphene citrate is given during the early follicular phase to ovulating women, an increase of LH and a milder enhancement of FSH can be seen

(Vandenberg & Yen, 1973). It seems that clomiphene increases the amplitude of the pulsatile discharge of gonadotropins from the pituitary. The exaggerated FSH levels in responsive patients probably stimulate the growth of a greater crop of follicles. These follicles, in the presence of increased LH levels, produce more estrogens than are synthesized in normal cycles. Estrogens enhance the pituitary response to GnRH and increase ovarian sensitivity to gonadotropins. Highly sensitized preovulatory follicles exposed to exaggerated gonadotropic stimulation are thus compelled to ovulate. The occupation of hypothalamic estrogen receptors by clomiphene is a time-limited process of rather short duration. A fair chance exists that, by the time ovarian follicles that are stimulated by the clomiphene-induced gonadotropin elevation reach the preovulatory stage, the hypothalamus is already free of clomiphene influence and ready to perceive the correct steroid signal. From this moment on, the events are regulated and controlled by the endogenous feedback mechanism within the hypothalamic-pituitary-ovarian axis. In inducing ovulation, clomiphene acts essentially as a primary gonadotropin releaser, creating the first push necessary for initiating the development of a set of follicles.

Antiestrogenic Effects on the Cervix and Endometrium

The antiestrogenic activity of clomiphene citrate and tamoxifen may exert an adverse influence on the endometrium, cervix and its mucus. This detrimental effect, due to the drug's competition for estrogen receptors on the uterine and cervical epithelium, is claimed to be one factor responsible for the discrepancy between the ovulation rate (70%) and the pregnancy rate (32%) in women receiving clomiphene citrate treatment. We have observed an antiestrogenic effect following clomiphene citrate treatment in several patients. An illustrative example of this effect in one of our patients is shown in Figure 5–4. The antiestrogenic effect on the cervical mucus, when present, is expressed by low cervical score which occurs despite the relatively high levels of estrogen in the circulation. In many patients given clomiphene, the cervical mucus does not exhibit any suppression. To understand this phenomenon, we must remember the antiestrogen effect on the hypothalamus which results in elevated FSH and LH levels. The elevated gonadotropin levels can cause multifollicular development, which in turn enhances estrogen production. The elevated estrogen levels, five to ten times higher than in normal cycles, sometimes mask the antiestrogen effect of clomiphene citrate and tamoxifen. In some instances the excessive estradiol concentration produced by a number of medium-sized follicles may induce an early or untimely estrogen-evoked LH surge which will induce luteinization prior to their full maturation. The antiestrogenic effect of CC on the endometrium is probably similar to that exerted by the drug upon the endocervical epithelium and may be explained by a similar mechanism.

Kokko et al. (1981) reported that administration of clomiphene citrate to untreated or estrogen-treated postmenopausal women results in progressive endometrial atrophy and a diminution of the endometrial concentrations of cytosolic estrogen and progesterone receptors.

It has been indeed suspected that some of the reasons for the discrepancy between the ovulation and pregnancy rates observed in infertile patients treated with CC lie in the reduced capability of the out-of-phase endometrium to receive and support the fertilized egg. It should, however, be remembered that the relatively high estrogen levels characteristic for the CC-induced cycles may probably effectively counteract the antiestrogenic action of CC in most women treated with this drug.

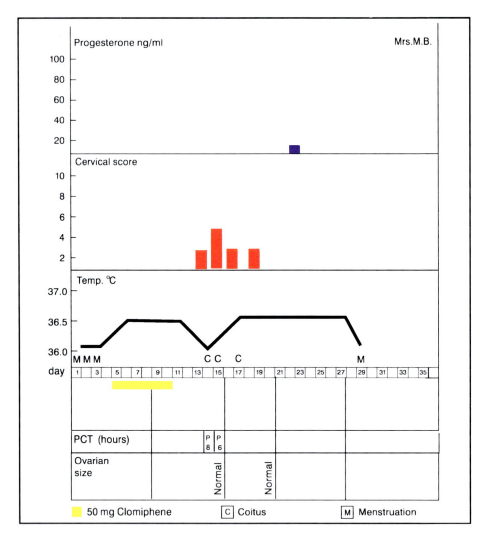

Fig. 5–4. Clomiphene therapy monitored by BBT, cervical score, and plasma progesterone. Note the significant suppression of the cervical score around the ovulation time and the corresponding poor postcoital tests.

Selection of Patients

Considering its mode of action, an antiestrogen such as clomiphene should be effective in patients having a hypothalamus capable of producing GnRH, a pituitary gland capable of response to GnRH, and an ovary containing follicles at various stages of development. Clomiphene should be used in patients with hypothalamic-pituitary dysfunction (WHO Group II) who lack the proper regulation within the hypothalamic-pituitary-ovarian axis. These infertile women probably have irregularities in the pulsatile secretion of GnRH, even though they do have fluctuating, detectable levels of gonadotropins and estrogens. They exhibit various types of menstrual disorders such as oligomenorrhea, regular or irregular cycles with absent or infrequent ovulation, luteal phase deficiencies, and amenorrhea with endogenous estrogenic activity. Clomiphene may also be used in treating PCO syndrome. However, although a high percentage of PCO patients may ovulate following treatment, they are at risk for multiple pregnancies and ovarian hyperstimulation. Patients with amenorrhea and low endogenous levels of estrogens (hypothalamic-pituitary failure, WHO Group I) are usually not responsive to clomiphene.

Treatment Schemes and Monitoring of Clomiphene Therapy

Dosage and Duration of Treatment

Clomiphene citrate is administered orally in 50 mg tablets. Most physicians advocate a short course/low dose therapy consisting of 50–100 mg of clomiphene daily for five to seven days. Higher daily doses or prolonged treatment may increase the incidence of complications without significantly improving the conception rate.

No well-defined dose-response relationship has been proven between the amount of clomiphene citrate administered and the level of gonadotropins secreted or between the dose of clomiphene and the incidence of ovulation. However, Shepard et al. (1979) found a correlation between body weight and the clomiphene dose required for ovulation, which provides a rationale for treating obese women with an initial dose of 100 mg.

Some patients will not ovulate when given 50 mg of clomiphene daily for five days but will respond to a higher dose of 75, 100, or 150 mg daily. It is our policy to begin the therapy with 50 mg of clomiphene citrate over a period of five to seven days, starting between the third to fifth day of spontaneous or induced bleeding. If no response is obtained, the dose is successively increased in subsequent treatments until 100 or 150 mg per day are given. If ovulation is not evoked at this dosage, combined clomiphene/hCG therapy may be attempted. The smallest effective clomiphene dose is continued for six cycles. One has to remember that a significant fraction of patients may conceive within three months following initiation of therapy. Patients who do not conceive after six apparently ovulatory, clomiphene-treatment cycles are thoroughly reinvestigated in order to diagnose previously undetected pathologies (male factor, well-hidden endometriotic foci and other mechanical factors, mild hyperandrogenicity, and thyroid dysfunction). Patients are also evaluated for possible clomiphene-induced infertility caused by its antiestrogenic effects. This effect may express itself by producing hostile cervical mucus or an endometrium unfavorable to implantation. Clomiphene may also evoke early and excessive estrogen secretion which may result in premature luteinization of follicles due to an untimely LH surge. In some women, the abnormal estrogen milieu may also produce abnormally high LH levels during the follicular phase, thus interfering with normal development of the follicle and maturation of the ovum. Patients who do not ovulate following clomiphene therapy should be offered hMG/hCG (FSH/hCG) therapy. This treatment may also be applied to patients who failed to conceive following clomiphene therapy and to those in whom the antiestrogenic effects of clomiphene could be responsible for conception failure. In the latter group, a combined clomiphene/high dose estrogen therapy may also be tried (Scharf et al. 1971; Seki et al. 1973; Insler et al. 1973a).

Monitoring of Therapy

In order to obtain optimal results, clomiphene therapy should be carefully monitored. Obviously, serial estimations of FSH, LH, estrogen, and progesterone levels provide the most detailed information on the patient's response to clomiphene. This method of monitoring is, however, too expensive and time consuming for the patient and presents too big a strain for the laboratory to be employed in standard treatment (even if very sophisticated laboratory service is available on a full time basis). Moreover, patients on clomiphene therapy have notoriously capricious responses to ovulation induction. Among these patients, even the most detailed data obtained in one treatment cycle are not necessarily applicable to another treatment course in the same patient. To be clinically useful, the method of monitoring clomiphene treatment should be able to give some indication as to whether the therapy provoked follicular development, if and when ovulation took place, and whether the corpus luteum was of proper quality and duration. Additional information of value can be provided by monitoring the quality and sperm penetrability of the cervical mucus. To be practicably applied in a busy fertility clinic, the method has to be inexpensive, rapid, and relatively easy to perform. In our clinic, clomiphene therapy is monitored by BBT records, by estimation of the cervical score (Insler et al. 1972) combined with postcoital tests, by sonographic measurements of follicular diameter and by blood progesterone assays. In practice, the monitoring of clomiphene treatment is carried out as follows. Patients are instructed to record daily BBT measurements. Clomiphene citrate is ingested in the prescribed dose each evening starting between the third and fifth day following initiation of menses and is continued for five to seven consecutive days. Between the fourth and sixth day after cessation of clomiphene ingestion, the patient is instructed to have sexual intercourse and to appear at the clinic two to ten hours thereafter. On this visit, a cervical mucus sample is taken, the cervical score is estimated, and a postcoital test is performed. At this stage, sonographic scans are also performed to assess the number and size of ovarian follicles. A careful vaginal examination is carried out. If the cervical score is 8 points or more, the postcoital test is at least fair, and at least one follicle exceeding in diameter 15 mm is present, the patient is instructed to have intercourse daily for the next two to three days. During the next visit five to six days later, the BBT record is evaluated and the patient is questioned about possible side effects indicative of hyperstimulation, such as weight gain, abdominal pain, nausea, and vomiting. If any of these symptoms are present, a vaginal examination is carried out, the size of the ovaries is carefully estimated, and an ultrasound scan is performed. Ovarian hyperstimulation, if present, is classified and treated in the same manner as that following gonadotropin therapy (see Chapter 7). Blood sampling for progesterone is scheduled for the sixth to eighth day following the temperature nadir preceding the sustained high temperature phase (Fig. 5-5).

In patients having a low cervical score (less than 8 points) and/or a poor or negative postcoital test and/or in whom no growing follicles are seen on sonography on the first visit, the examination is repeated daily until either the score becomes 8 points, a sustained BBT rise and the disappearance of a previously seen large follicle indicate that ovulation has taken place, or neither of these events appear during 12 days following the cessation of clomiphene. The examination has to be carried out daily, at least in the first treatment cycle, since the cervical crypts may be freed from the antiestrogenic action of clomiphene only for a very brief period around ovulation, during which it is essential to examine the mucus.

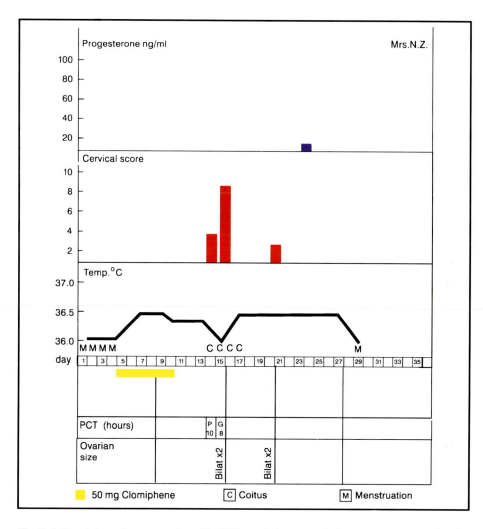

Fig. 5-5. Clomiphene therapy monitored by BBT, cervical score, and plasma progesterone estimation. The cervical score was very low (4 points) one day before the temperature nadir, increased to 10 points around the time of presumed ovulation, and became negative 5 days later. The postcoital test (PCT) was poor (P) one day before presumed ovulation and good (G) on the day of temperature nadir, corresponding with the high cervical score. Ovulation was indicated by the biphasic temperature pattern and plasma progesterone of 20 ng/ml.

Treatment with clomiphene (50 mg for five days) may fail even in a patient belonging to the appropriate group. Among the 75% who will ovulate, only 50% will become pregnant. Many women will ovulate in response to clomiphene doses higher than 50 mg. There are reports that larger doses administered for a duration exceeding five days may also induce ovulation.

It has been shown that obese women require higher doses of clomiphene in order to successfully compete with elevated estrogens for hypothalamic receptors.

Results of Clomiphene Therapy

It is customary to assess the results of clomiphene therapy by calculating ovulation and pregnancy rates. These parameters are excellent for estimating the efficacy of clomiphene treatment in well-defined groups of patients. However, when one tries to draw some general conclusions from scanning the literature and comparing the results obtained in various groups of patients treated at different centers, the complete lack of uniformity in the classification of anovulatory patients becomes an almost insurmountable obstacle. For this reason, Table 5-2 presents the results of clomiphene treatment as reported by various authors without any attempt at classification, comparison or discussion. One fact seems to be obvious from this Table.

TABLE 5-2. Ovulation and Pregnancy Rates following Clomiphene Therapy as reported by various Authors

Authors	Year	No. of Patients	Ovulation Rate (%)	Pregnancy Rate (%)
Whitelaw et al.	1964	37	72.9	45.9
Pildes	1965	36	50.0	11.1
Kistner	1965	50	96.0	26.0
Kase et al.	1967	81	60.5	25.9
Rabau et al.	1967	101	62.6	33.6
Seegar-Jones & Moraes-Ruehsen	1967	73	83.0	30.1
Spellacy & Cohen	1967	35	80.0	20.0
MacGregor et al.	1968	6 714	70.0	32.7
MacLeod et al.	1970	118	77.0	31.1
Greenblatt & Dalla Pria	1971	257	77.0	–
Murray & Osmond-Clarke	1971	328	66.5	25.0
Evans & Townsend	1976	145	80.7	56.0
Gorlitzky et al.	1978	122	56.6	36.9
Gysler et al.	1982	428	85.3	42.8
Hammond et al.	1983	159	86.1	49.0

Although most authors reported the ovulation rate to be 70% or higher, the mean pregnancy rate reported in this compilation of 8,584 patients was 33.1%. The discrepancy between ovulation rate and pregnancy rate may be due to luteal phase inadequacy following clomiphene-induced cycles (Seegar-Jones et al. 1970), abnormal tubal transport (Whitelaw et al. 1970), cervical mucus hostility (Figuerora Casas et al. 1970; Insler et al. 1973a), or ovum entrapment within the follicle.

Follicular luteinization (Kase et al. 1967) may also occur and mimic ovulation as far as BBT measurements and progesterone levels are concerned.

About one half of those women who eventually ovulate will do so in response to the dose of 100 mg. Only a few will require higher doses. Patients with anovulatory cycles or oligomenorrhea seem to ovulate and conceive more readily than those with amenorrhea (93% vs. 59%) (Gysler et al. 1982). Most patients conceive during the first three ovulatory cycles; a small group will become pregnant when treatment is continued for longer periods. Pregnancy rate per ovulatory cycle in otherwise normal women is approximately 32%.

Outcome of Pregnancy

The incidence of multiple pregnancy in clomiphene citrate-treated patients is approximately 8 to 9 times higher than in spontaneous pregnancy. There is no a significant difference in the entire outcome compared to spontaneous pregnancies. Summing up 3,486 pregnancies from the literature (1969–1983), we found an abortion rate of 17%, with reported ranges from 8.9% (Gorlitzky et al. 1978), to as high as 22.8% (Murray & Osmond-Clarke, 1971). Kurachi et al. (1983) reported the outcome of 1,034 pregnancies following clomiphene citrate therapy and found an abortion rate of 14.2%.

The cause of the 17% mean abortion rate is still unknown. It is possible that at least some abortions may be due to corpus luteum insufficiency indicated by a short luteal phase, which often follows clomiphene-induced ovulation (Seegar-Jones et al. 1970; Murray & Osmond-Clarke, 1971). The possibility that the antiestrogenic action of clomiphene citrate upon the endometrium may interfere with implantation of the fertilized ovum is negated by the finding of histologically normal endometrium in patients in whom hormonal indices showed that ovulation had taken place. It should be pointed out that higher abortion rates have been shown to follow almost every kind of infertility treatment, including tubal surgery and artificial insemination. The outcome of pregnancies in Kurachi's sample included 0.5% extrauterine pregnancies, 0.1% hydatidiform moles, 5.9% premature births, and 79.3% full term births. These impressive data indicate that there is hardly any difference between the outcome of pregnancies following spontaneous ovulation and clomiphene citrate-treated cycles.

Incremental and Combined Therapy

Incremental Clomiphene Therapy

O'Herlihy et al. (1981) used large doses of clomiphene to induce ovulation. He treated the so-called clomiphene failures in a continuous manner until follicular maturation was attained. To find the effective dose (i.e. the amount of clomiphene required to cause follicular growth), he increased the dose every five days by 50 mg while measuring estrogen levels and monitoring follicular development by ultra-sound. The initial dose was 50 mg per day, and the final dose never exceeded 250 mg per day. When follicular development reached 18–19 mm, an ovulatory dose of hCG was administered. This treatment resulted in ovulation in 70% of women who did not respond to conventional clomiphene therapy. The pregnancy rate was 27%.

Clomiphene /hCG Therapy

The most popular combination seems to be sequential clomiphene/hCG therapy (Fig. 5-6). Some patients show only a partial response to clomiphene, with an indication of progressive follicular development but no ensuing ovulation. Clomiphene apparently exerts its primary action in these women, causing the release of GnRH and sensitizing the pituitary and the ovaries to their respective stimulants. The initial gonadotropin elevation can be readily observed in such patients, and evidence of follicular development is found in rising estrogen levels and/or by ultrasound scans. However, the endogenous feedback mechanism responsible for the preovulatory LH surge is not properly activated, and consequently the midcycle LH peak may be entirely absent, inadequate, or ill timed. Some authors believe that the increased

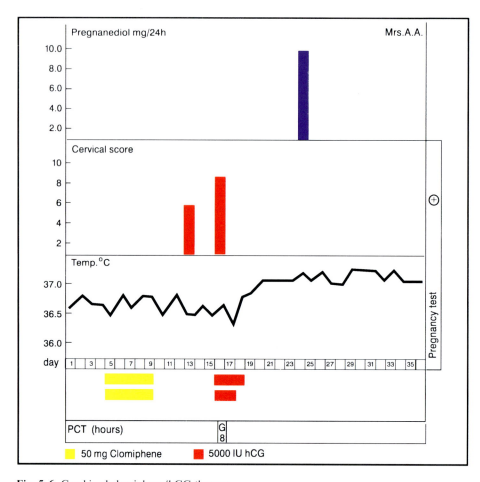

Fig. 5-6. Combined clomiphene/hCG therapy.

amount of inhibitory substances released by the supranormal number of mature follicles inhibits the LH surge (Schenken & Hodgen, 1983). In such cases, hCG should be administered to induce ovulation.

The pregnancy rate of the clomiphene/hCG regime has been found disappointing by some authors (Swyer et al. 1975), but in any case it is not very high. This might be due to untimely administration of hCG, which causes atresia or luteinization (Williams & Hodgen, 1980). To determine when to initiate hCG administration, O'Herlihy and his coworkers (1982) used ultrasound scanning to detect the presence of a mature follicle. With this method, they achieved 14 ovulations from 21 previously nonovulatory women. Four of the seven who did not conceive were found by laparoscopy to have endometriosis.

We use combined clomiphene/hCG treatment in patients who show an adequate ovarian response but do not ovulate when treated with clomiphene alone at the dose level of at least 100 mg per day. The combined treatment is carried out as follows.

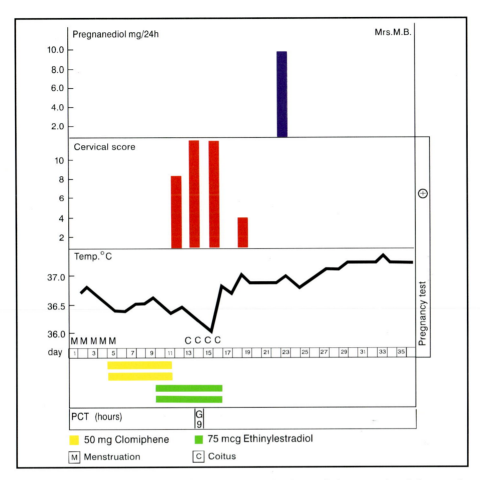

Fig. 5-7. Combined clomiphene/estrogen therapy. Ethinyl estradiol was continued for one day following the temperature rise. The cervical score around the time of ovulation was 12 points, indicating that the estrogen was able to counteract the suppressive action of clomiphene upon the cervical epithelium. Ovulation was indicated by biphasic temperature pattern, high plasma progesterone level, and confirmed by ensuing pregnancy.

Clomiphene citrate (100 mg daily) is started on the third to fifth day of the menstrual cycle and continued for five days. The patient is examined daily from the fourth day following cessation of clomiphene. Whenever the cervical score reaches or exceeds 8 points, an ultrasound scan is performed. If a mature follicle(s) – greater than 18 mm – is demonstrated, 10,000 IU of hCG are administered.

Clomiphene / Estrogen Therapy

Clomiphene citrate, acting as an antiestrogen, severely depresses the vaginal epithelium and, to a lesser degree, the endocervical crypts. Since multifollicular development is induced under clomiphene therapy the elevated estrogen levels usually override this effect. However, in some cases the antiestrogen effect results in thick, tenacious mucus which may prevent conception by hindering sperm from migrating through the cervical canal. The discrepancy between the ovulation rate and the conception rate following clomiphene therapy may, in some of these cases, be due to the drug's suppressive effect on the uterine cervix. In such cases, combined clomiphene/estrogen therapy may significantly improve the results.

The combined clomiphene/estrogen therapy is executed as follows: Clomiphene is given for five or six consecutive days starting on the third to fifth day following spontaneous or induced bleeding. On the last two days of clomiphene administration, ethinyl estradiol is added daily until the shift of BBT has occurred. The effective dose is usually between 50 and 150 micrograms of ethinyl estradiol (EE) or an equivalent dose of another estrogen preparation. This amount is capable of producing a good cervical response (a cervical score of more than 8 points) within seven to nine days of administration in some women. Patients are then requested to have intercourse daily until the increase in BBT measurement indicates that ovulation has occurred (Fig. 5–7).

Clomiphene Citrate and hMG

The rationale of clomiphene citrate followed by hMG is the utilization of the former to increase FSH in the initial phase (follicular recruitment and selection) and to maintain adequate FSH levels by administration of hMG during the follicular growth phase. This method has found wide acceptance in in vitro fertilization programs and has also been used in ovulation induction in anovulatory patients mainly to reduce the amount of hMG needed, and thus the cost of therapy (March et al. 1976).

Kistner (1976) found a pregnancy rate of 28%, and Robertson et al. (1977) reported a pregnancy rate of 49%. It is interesting to note that the latter sample demonstrated a high level of hyperstimulation, as evidenced by 2 sets of triplets and 3 sets of quadruplets in their series.

The clomiphene citrate/hMG treatment scheme is as follows: On the fifth through ninth days after induced or spontaneous bleeding, the normogonadotropic patient receives 100 mg of clomiphene citrate daily. From the eighth day onwards, hMG is administered. The patient is carefully monitored by estrogen determinations and ultrasound visualization of the growing follicle(s). This will help to determine if and when the ovulatory dose of hCG should be administered and to reduce the incidence of hyperstimulation and multiple pregnancies. When estrogen reaches preovulatory levels in the presence of one to three follicles with a diameter of 18–22 mm, 5,000–10,000 IU of hCG are administered.

Complications of Clomiphene Therapy

Complications of clomiphene therapy may be roughly divided into two groups: (1) untoward effects of ovarian stimulation and induction of ovulation, and (2) side effects of the drug itself. The former group includes ovarian hyperstimulation. The administration of clomiphene citrate may cause the development of large multiple ovarian cysts. Sometimes this finding may be accompanied by severe abdominal pain, nausea, vomiting, ascites, and hydrothorax. Since the pathophysiology, symptoms, and treatment of hyperstimulation syndrome are similar, whether they are caused by clomiphene therapy or by other ovulation-inducing therapies, the syndrome will be discussed in detail in the section on complications of gonadotropic treatment (see Chapter 7).

The incidence of severe hyperstimulation syndrome (Grade 3) is low following clomiphene administration. Ovarian enlargement accompanied by some abdominal pain is, however, encountered quite frequently. Kistner (1975), reviewing treatment records of 5,836 patients treated with clomiphene, found ovarian enlargement in 13.8% of all cases. However, when short course therapy (not exceeding seven days) was used, the incidence of ovarian enlargement was reduced to 5.4% in single course and to 7.8% in multiple course therapy. This is consistent with the 5.1% hyperstimulation rate reported by Gysler et al. (1982). Murray & Osmond-Clarke (1971) encountered painful ovarian enlargement in only 2 women of the 328 treated with 100–200 mg of clomiphene citrate daily for four days. Rust et al. (1974) observed the appearance of ovarian cysts in 7 of 105 patients (6.7%) receiving clomiphene doses of up to 250 mg daily for up to five days. Only one of these women received 150 mg of clomiphene daily, and none received a higher dose. It should be noted that the sensitivity of the ovary may vary from cycle to cycle, and that the occurrence of hyperstimulation does not necessarily mean that the ovary will overreact in subsequent treatment cycles (Bailer et al. 1980).

The preceding data indicate that, when considering ovarian enlargement, the length of therapy is more important than the dose of clomiphene. Doses of up to 200 mg per day, confined to four to six days, keep the incidence of hyperstimulation within reasonable limits. Since the reaction of any patient to clomiphene is unpredictable, it is always advisable to begin with the lowest dose (50 mg daily) and then to increase it gradually in subsequent cycles. Ovarian cysts developing after clomiphene treatment usually resolve spontaneously within a few weeks. During this period, clomiphene should not be administered.

Apart from the complications directly related to ovarian stimulation, several side effects of clomiphene citrate due to the pharmacologic action of the drug on various tissues and organs have been observed. Hot flashes are quite common, appearing in about 10% of the patients. Although resembling those observed during menopause, hot flashes caused by clomiphene are probably not due to the antiestrogenic effect of the drug, since they are not ameliorated by concomitant administration of estrogen. Nausea, vomiting, and breast discomfort occur in about 2% of the patients and may be attributed to the relative hyperestrogenism caused by clomiphene. Mild visual disturbances are noted in 1.6%, skin reactions such as dermatitis or urticaria in 0.6%, and hair loss in 0.4%. All of the above side effects are reversible and disappear a few days after cessation of clomiphene ingestion.

Congenital Malformations

Various studies on large series of patients who delivered after clomiphene treatment do not report a significantly elevated malformation rate. Kurachi et al. (1983) compared the malformation rate between 931 infants born after clomiphene citrate treatment and 30,033 infants born with no treatment at the time of the study. He found no significant differences between the incidence or type of malformations. However, individual case reports showed neural tube defects and Down's syndrome, raising the question whether pregnancies following clomiphene therapy should be screened with alphafetoprotein and cytogenetic studies. Since in about two thirds of DES-exposed offspring some cervical or uterine anomalies have been noted, and since clomiphene is structurally related to DES, clomiphene should be carefully avoided if pregnancy is suspected.

Merrel-National Laboratories reported 158 pregnancies in which the mothers received clomiphene during pregnancy. In 7 of these 158 pregnancies, 5 babies had minor and 3 had major malformations.

Final conclusions regarding the possible teratogenic effects of clomiphene on the development of the mullerian ducts and on the later function of the reproductive organs will have to be delayed until surveys on postpubertal offspring following clomiphene therapy have been concluded.

6. PROLACTIN-INHIBITING AGENTS

INTRODUCTION

It has been apparent for a long time that inappropriate prolactin secretion may be of clinical importance in humans. However, significant progress in this area was made possible only after specific assays of human prolactin were made available for clinical use. Friesen et al. (1972) showed that primate pituitaries synthesize and secrete prolactin and that this hormone may be immunologically distinguished and separated from growth hormone. Primate prolactin is immunologically related to prolactin from other species. Prolactin was characterized (Lewis et al. 1971) and purified (Hwang et al. 1972) and radio-immuno-assays for the measurement of prolactin levels in serum have been developed (Hwang et al. 1972). This has contributed to the elucidation of the control mechanism of the hormone.

Human prolactin is a single-chain polypeptide hormone containing 198 amino acids and with a molecular weight of 22,500 daltons (Shome & Parlow, 1977). It is secreted mainly by the anterior pituitary. However, convincing evidence has been presented to support the view that the decidua is also a significant source of prolactin (Golander et al. 1978). At least three different radio-immuno-assayable forms of circulating prolactin can be detected: monomeric prolactin which is the native and biologically active form, big prolactin (molecular weight 50,000 daltons), and big-big prolactin which probably represents aggregates of the monomeric forms (Benveniste et al. 1979).

Big-big prolactin appears to be biologically inactive, and recent preliminary reports have described women with big-big hyperprolactinemia and normal menstrual cycles. Other forms of biologically potent prolactin with no immuno-reactivity have been described (Whittaker, 1981). Apparently, with different states of pituitary activity and/or certain pathological states, there is a release of different prolactin forms.

ETIOLOGY OF HYPERPROLACTINEMIA

The existence of galactorrhea-amenorrhea syndromes has been known for more than a century, although their endocrine etiology was not elucidated until more than a hundred years later (Frommel, 1882; Argonz & Del Castillo, 1953; Forbes et al. 1954).

Hyperprolactinemia may be caused by several functional and anatomical mechanisms:

1. Hypothalamic diseases such as encephalitis or meningitis and granulomatous or tumoral infiltration can cause hyperprolactinemia by a mechanism of decreased hypothalamic dopamine secretion;
2. Stalk lesions which interfere with the transport of dopamine to the portal system and to the anterior pituitary can cause hyperprolactinemia by the same mechanism, namely, decrease in tonic inhibition of pituitary prolactin secretion;
3. Pituitary tumors can secrete prolactin because of adenoma formation by the lactotroph cells (prolactinomas). Other pituitary hypersecreting tumors are also associated with hyperprolactinemia. 20–30 % of cases of acromegaly (Corenblum

TABLE 6-1. Drugs stimulating Prolactin Release

Neuroleptics
Phenothiazines (Chlorpromazine)
Butyrophenones (Haloperidol)
Diphenyl-butylpiperidine (Pimozide)
Sulpiride (Dogmatyl)

Antidepressants
Dibenzepin derivatives (Imipramine)

Antihypertensives
α-Methyldopa (Aldomet)
Reserpine (Serpasil)

Hormones
TRH
Estrogens

Others
Metoclopramide
Cimetidine (H-2-receptor histamine antagonist)
Timolol
Yohimbine
Piperoxan
Morphine
Methadone

et al. 1976) and 5–10% of cases of Cushing's disease are hyperprolactinemic. Usually, especially in acromegaly, there is evidence of a mixed endocrine tumor also containing lactotroph cells. In some of the cases, as demonstrated by hyperprolactinemia in non-functional pituitary tumors, the tumor size by itself may cause changes in the portal blood supply which, in turn, may result in decreased dopamine levels, producing hyperprolactinemia (Frank et al. 1977);

4. Chest wall and breast stimulation which activate the normal nursing reflex in the puerperium can cause hyperprolactinemia in certain pathological states, e.g. following thoracotomy, mastectomy, herpes zoster infections of the chest wall, dermatomes, and chest wall burns (Herman et al. 1981);

5. Various pharmacological agents can cause hyperprolactinemia by various mechanisms (Table 6-1). Reserpine and methyldopa act by depleting hypothalamic dopamine. Phenothiazines, butyrophenones, sulpiride, and metoclopramide all produce hyperprolactinemia by dopamine receptor blockade (Del Pozzo et al. 1976). Estrogens directly affect the ability of lactotrophs to synthesize and secrete prolactin by modulating the response to various stimuli (Raymond et al. 1978);

6. Primary hypothyroidism can produce hyperprolactinemia. The mechanism is not yet clear but a decrease in hypothalamic dopamine and/or an increase in hypothalamic thyroid-releasing hormone (TRH) secretion have been suggested (Feek et al. 1980; Contreras et al. 1981). Adequate thyroid hormone replacement results in a restoration of prolactin levels toward normal;

7. Hyperprolactinemia in chronic renal failure was attributed to the reduced metabolic clearance of prolactin and to the increase in its production rate (Frohman et al. 1981).

HYPERPROLACTINEMIA AND ANOVULATION

It has been demonstrated that excessive secretion of prolactin can cause amenorrhea with or without galactorrhea and that it may also lead to anovulation or disturbed corpus luteum function. Mild hyperprolactinemia has also been found in 18–27% of patients with polycystic ovarian disease. Lactotroph cell stimulation by constant and excessive estrogen secretion is a logical cause for this phenomenon. It may now be safe to presume that, in hyperprolactinemic women, the pulsatility of GnRH secretion is disturbed, leading to disarrayed gonadotropin secretion and consequently to the functional ovarian disturbances described above. Depending on the relative concentrations of prolactin, the LH surge may be completely neutralized, resulting in anovulation, or it may be partially inhibited, resulting in corpus luteum insufficiency. It has been shown that the positive feedback effect of estrogen on LH secretion is suppressed in women with hyperprolactinemia (Nyboe Andersen et al. 1982) and that pulsatile secretion of LH was either discontinued or reduced in amplitude during periods of maximal prolactin secretion (Boyar et al. 1975). Discontinuation or impairment of pulsatile release of LH was also reported by Bohnet et al. (1976).

Moult et al. (1982) showed that performing bromocriptine therapy in women with hyperprolactinemic amenorrhea restored the normal rate of LH pulsatility. Leyendecker et al. (1980) reported success in inducing ovulation in hyperprolactinemic women by pulsatile administration of LH-RH, despite persistent elevation of prolactin concentrations. This report provides convincing evidence of the mechanism involved in the impairment of fertility in hyperprolactinemic states.

Elevated prolactin levels may also cause ovarian refractoriness to gonadotropins. Thorner et al. (1975) have observed resistance to the effect of exogenous gonadotropins in hyperprolactinemic women, which disappeared after prolactin levels were lowered. Others have shown the same phenomenon of ovarian refractoriness to exogenous gonadotropins in the physiologically hyperprolactinemic state of the puerperium. In addition, McNatty et al. (1977) have shown experimentally that prolactin may exert a specific effect on ovarian steroidogenesis in vitro, and that there appears to be an inverse relationship between prevailing prolactin levels and the steroidogenic potential of the follicular cells.

Kaupilla et al. (1982), using both ultrasonographic and endocrinological investigations, demonstrated that metoclopramide-induced hyperprolactinemia interferes with follicular maturation. They found irregularities in follicular size, selection of the dominant follicle, and follicular and corpus luteum steroidogenesis in women treated with this drug.

In contrast, other authors have suggested that prolactin has no direct effect upon the ovary, since stimulation of the ovaries of hyperprolactinemic amenorrheic patients with gonadotropins has induced ovulation and pregnancy. Lunenfeld et al. (1970) were able to show that patients with amenorrhea and galactorrhea could be efficiently treated with human gonadotropins (hMG); moreover, the required doses were lower than in amenorrheic women without galactorrhea.

CONTROL OF PROLACTIN SECRETION

During the last few years, various pharmacological agents have been used in an attempt to reduce abnormally high prolactin levels. In order to understand the mechanisms of action of these drugs, as well as the pathogenesis in iatrogenic hyperprolactinemia and the rationale behind the dynamic tests for prolactin secretion, some knowledge of the neuroendocrine regulation of this hormone is necessary. Prolactin is unique among pituitary hormones in being under predominantly inhibitory control from the hypothalamus. There is no specific end-organ secretion mediating feedback control. Instead, a substance termed prolactin-inhibitory factor (PIF) is liberated by the hypothalamus into the portal vessels and exerts inhibitory control of prolactin secretion. This fact is clearly manifested by the fact that pituitary stalk section causes hyperprolactinemia and a decrease of all the other pituitary hormones.

The consensus remains that the prolactin secretion inhibitory property is definitely linked to the stimulation of dopamine (DA) receptors on the lactotrophs' cell membrane (Flueckiger et al. 1976). This concept is substantiated by the demonstration that dopamine inhibits prolactin secretion both in lactotroph tissue culture and in in vivo experiments in animals and humans (MacLeod et al. 1970) and by the fact that many pharmacological agents capable of blocking dopamine receptors can cause iatrogenic hyperprolactinemia.

A number of substances are known to have PIF activity. The amino acid GABA (gamma-Amino-butyric-acid), found in significant concentrations within the median eminence, is one such substance. Moreover, GABA receptors are found on pituitary cell membranes (Racagni et al. 1979; Grandison et al. 1982). Although the exact physiological role of GABA in regulating prolactin secretion remains to be elucidated, it is clear that it does not act via the dopaminergic system. Other substances like catecholamines, cholinergic agonists, and prolactin itself act as inhibitory factors via the dopaminergic system of the tuberoinfundibular tract.

Specific prolactin-releasing factor (PRF) was demonstrated clearly using hypothalamic extracts (Valverde et al. 1972). TRH (Tashjian et al. 1971), serotonin (Wehrenberg et al. 1980), opioids, GnRH (Denef, 1981), vasoactive intestinal peptide (VIP) (Ruberg et al. 1978), vasopressin (Shin, 1982), substance P (Vijayan & McCann, 1979), and estradiol (Vician et al. 1979) were shown to exert PRF-like activity. Some of these substances, especially estrogens, may also act as modulators of the response of lactotroph cells to various prolactin-releasing stimuli (Raymond et al. 1978).

SELECTION OF PATIENTS FOR TREATMENT WITH PROLACTIN-INHIBITING AGENTS

In the evaluation of infertile patients with menstrual disorders, prolactin determination is recommended as one of the first laboratory tests. Seventy five per cent of the galactorrheic amenorrheic patients and about 15% of all other women with menstrual cycle disorders have various degrees of hyperprolactinemia.

In principle, all infertile patients exhibiting hyperprolactinemia (in our laboratory, above 15 ng/ml) will benefit from the inhibition of prolactin secretion. Hyperprolactinemic patients may exhibit amenorrhea, anovulation, luteal insufficiency, or other menstrual cycle disorders. Some of them will also exhibit galactorrhea. Before deciding on therapeutic strategy, the etiology of hyperprolactinemia must be assessed. Stress, iatrogenic causes, hypothyroidism, and chronic renal failure should be ruled out. If a space-occupying lesion of the sella turcica region is observed, its extension into the supra- and parasellar space must be assessed.

Four general criteria for detecting the presence of a pituitary prolactin-secreting tumor are now generally accepted. These include radiological evidence of a pituitary lesion, elevated prolactin levels, and visual field alteration.

The radiological classification of prolactinomas, which is widely accepted today, employs the criteria proposed by Hardy (1980): grade 0 (enclosed adenoma) can only be detected by prolactin measurements; grade I (microadenoma $\geq$ 10 mm in diameter) may show slight sellar erosion or deformation; grade II is a more advanced lesion with or without suprasellar extension; and grades III and IV (invasive tumors), are localized or diffuse with para- or suprasellar extension.

An enlarged pituitary fossa can be diagnosed from a plain skull radiograph, but patients with a microadenoma generally have a sella of normal size. The asymmetrical bulging of the sella floor in these patients is revealed only by thin-cut tomography. A CT-scan with the addition of contrast materials will show a microadenoma larger than 6–8 mm reaching the sella entrance. In addition, a CT-scan enables visualization of any extension of an adenoma into the supra- and parasellar space.

The refinement of CT-scanning, using the generation of tomograms with higher resolution power and the introduction of nuclear magnetic resonance technology (Hawkes et al. 1983), enables the direct demonstration of much smaller microadenomas. Pneumoencephalography is indicated only if an empty sella is suspected, and cerebral angiography is required if a carotid aneurysm has to be excluded.

If the pituitary neoplasm extends into the suprasellar area, compression of the optic nerve pathways can occur, leading to visual field defects, loss of vision, and, occasionally, optic nerve atrophy. Growth into the sphenoid sinus does not lead to clinical symptoms. Because most patients with suspected pituitary neoplasm are usually unaware of any visual impairment, it is important to carry out visual field examination. Bitemporal hemianopsia is the most typical sign (50% of cases), though other defects, such as central or nasal scotomas, can also occur. In a severe chiasma syndrome, pallor of the optic disc or complete atrophy of the papilla can be seen. Papilledema is only observed when the adenoma causes ventricular obstruction as it reaches the foramen of Monro. Parasellar extension can cause extraocular muscle palsies, such as ptosis, mydriasis, and diplopia, mainly through involvement of the third, fourth, and sixth cranial nerves. This is seen only in patients with very large adenomas or as an effect of pituitary apoplexy.

Today, most clinicians agree that the treatment of choice for pituitary tumors with supra- or parasellar extension requires surgical therapy at some stage. In all other patients suffering from hyperprolactimenia and its functional consequences, medical therapy is sufficient and effective. It should, however, be remembered that if the therapy is aimed at achieving ovulation and conception, induced pregnancy may cause an expansion of the pituitary tumor and lead to visual field defects and/or pituitary apoplexy. The reported incidence of these complication is as high as 35% in patients with macroadenomas but only 5% in patients with microadenomas (Gemzell & Wang, 1979; Bergh et al. 1978).

MEDICAL TREATMENT OF HYPERPROLACTINEMIA

Bromocriptine

Bromocriptine is an ergot derivative structurally resembling dopamine (Fig. 6-1).

After oral administration, 40-90% of the dose is absorbed from the gastrointestinal tract (Mehta & Tolis, 1979). Peak plasma levels occur 3 to 4 hours after oral administration (Fig. 6-2).

High plasma levels remain for several hours, the circulating half-life being 4 to 8 hours (Perkes, 1977; Thorner et al. 1980). Recently, bromocriptine microspheres have been made available. After being injected deep intragluteally, the bromocriptine content is released over 6 - 8 weeks (Lancranjan et al. 1987). Furthermore, a new long-acting bromocriptine was developed for monthly injections. In vivo experiments showed that the mass degradation of the polymer started after about 14 days and was nearly complete after 52 days.

Bromocriptine is metabolized extensively, especially in the liver, to at least 30 excretory products (Mehta & Tolis, 1979). The biological activity of the metabolites is unknown. More than 70% of the metabolized drug is excreted in the feces and only a small part is excreted in the urine (Perkes, 1977; Thorner et al. 1980). The drug is extremely hydrophilic and it crosses the blood brain barrier.

In the central nervous system, bromocriptine has a dual effect on dopamine metabolism. First, it acts as a direct, potent dopamine agonist on the dopamine receptor system of the pituitary gland. Bromocriptine binds to pituitary dopamine receptors (Caron et al. 1978) and inhibits spontaneous prolactin secretion and prolactin secretion stimulated by TSH (Mashiter et al. 1977). Second, bromocriptine decreases dopamine turnover in the hypothalamic tuberoinfundibular neurons resulting in higher concentration of dopamine in the hypothalamic-pituitary portal system (Hokfelt & Fuxe, 1972).

Bromocriptine may inhibit adenylate cyclase activity and reduce cellular cAMP content. The effects of bromocriptine on tumoral lactotrophs appears to be antitumoral. It decreases both RNA and DNA production, causing ultrastructural changes, particularly a decrease in cytoplasmatic and nuclear areas (Lloyd et al. 1975; Basseti et al. 1984). This effect apparently requires the presence of dopamine receptors on the tumor cells.

Monitoring of Treatment with Bromocriptine

Bromocriptine therapy should be initiated with a daily dose of 1.25 mg bromocriptine administered with food at bedtime. If the drug is well tolerated, within three days the dosage is increased to 1.25 mg b.i.d. After three additional days, the dosage is increased to 2.5 mg b.i.d. Five days later a prolactin determination is carried out. If prolactin levels are still high, the gradual dosage increase is continued until a therapeutically-effective dosage is reached. Therapeutically-effective dosage is defined as the dosage that results in menstruation, biphasic temperature curves, prolactin levels of 7-12 ng/ml, and luteal phase progesterone levels over 8 mg/ml (Fig. 6-3).

If after six months the patient has not conceived, a re-evaluation of the infertile couple is advised and further therapy discussed.

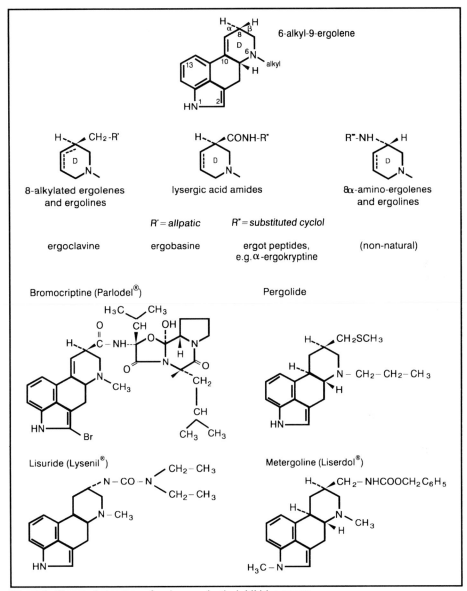

Fig. 6–1. Chemical structure of various prolactin-inhibiting agents.

Results of Treatment and Assessment of Complications

Since the introduction of bromocriptine in the early 1970's, literature on clinical experience with the drug has expanded exponentially. All reports agree about the very high effectiveness of bromocriptine in lowering prolactin levels, regardless of the etiology. In most of the responding cases, the sequence of events is usually as follows: Prolactin levels are normalized, GnRH pulsatility is restored followed by normal

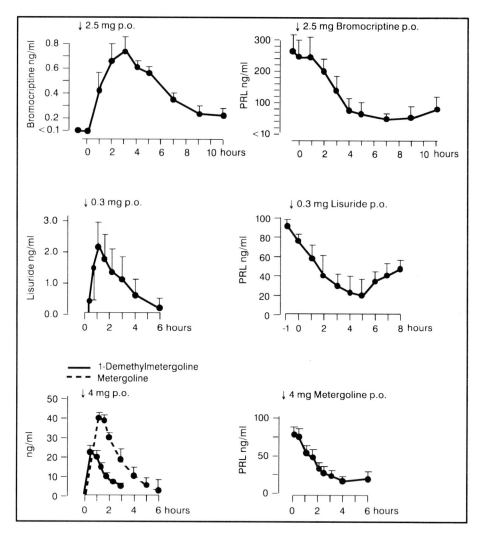

Fig. 6–2. Correlation between the increase and decrease of prolactin-inhibiting agents in blood and prolactin levels in hyperprolactinemic patients. (From: Data supplied by pharmaceutical companies: Sandoz, Schering and Farmitalia.)

dynamics of gonadotropin secretion, galactorrhea disappears, menstruation re-appears and, following some anovulatory or corpus luteum-deficient cycles, regular ovulatory cycles are re-established.

Bergh et al. (1978b) reported that among 42 hyperprolactinemic women with secondary amenorrhea, 21 patients conceived out of 22 who attempted to become pregnant. The prolactin levels decreased towards normal in all women, and ovulation returned after an average of 5.5 weeks. One interesting observation was that defective luteal function was observed during the first ovulatory cycle in 51% of the women, while 90% had a normal luteal phase after the second ovulation. The abortion rate was 22%. Table 6–2 lists results in terms of ovulation and pregnancy rates.

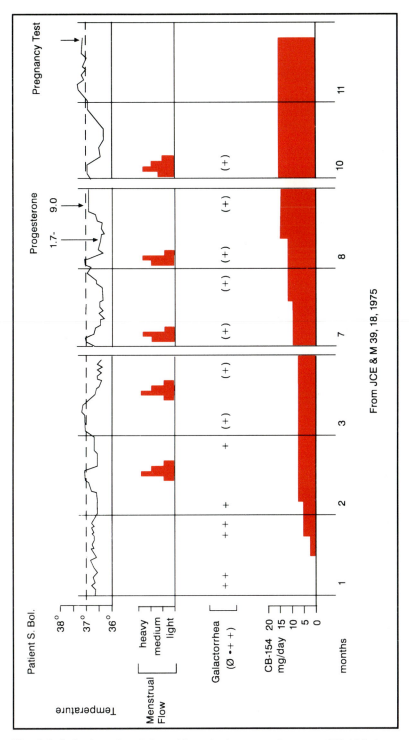

Fig. 6–3. Induction of ovulation with prolactin-suppressing agent (CB-154) in a patient with amenorrhea-galactorrhea syndrome.

TABLE 6–2. Results of Treatment of Hyperprolactinemia by Bromocriptine

Authors Year	Patients treated	Pro- lactin sup- pressed	Im- proved Galactor- rhea	Return of Menses	Ovula- tion	Preg- nancy
Thorner et al 1974	17	17	17	14	NR	2
Spark et al. 1976	15	15	15	14	14	4
Kleinberg et al. 1977	11	11	7	8	NR	2
Wiebe et al. 1977	13	11	13	10	11	3
Thorner & Besser 1977	70	60	NR	63	NR	37
Badano et al. 1977	30	23	21	17	17	7
Mroueh & Siller-Khodr 1977	28	19	19	19	17	9
Pepperell et al. 1977	20	20	16	20	20	14
Gomez et al. 1978	3	3	3	3	3	3
Bergh et al. 1978	29	26	NR	28	28	24
March et al. 1979	10	8	8	9	9	3
Bennink 1979	20	18	12	20	20	15
Scrabanek et al. 1980	33		20	20	NR	25
Crosignani et al. 1982	115	NR	NR	NR	64	44
DeBeranl & DeVillamizar 1982	18	3	NR	16	16	8
Corenblum & Taylor, 1983	20	25	NR	25	25	11
Cumulative*	468	259/320	151/200	286/353	278/337	211

NR = Not reported
* Cumulative values were calculated using the reports that included pertinent data (i. e. prolactin suppression is expressed „259/320"; since the reports of Scrabanek et al. and Crosignani lack these data, thus reducing the number of patients available for calculation to 320)

A multi-center surveillance program on pregnancies in women treated with bromocriptine provided information on the outcome of 1,410 pregnancies (Turkalj et al. 1982). The rate of spontaneous abortion was calculated to be 11.37%, corresponding well to normal controls. Ectopic pregnancies were reported in 12 patients and hydatidiform moles in three. The rate of multiple pregnancies was 2.9% (one triplet birth and 28 twin births), which is somewhat higher than in the normal population. Severe malformations were seen in 1% and minor abnormalities were detected in 2.5% of the infants. These rates are within normal limits. Of the 1,236 children born, 212 had been followed up for 3–36 months, and there was no indication that intrauterine exposure to bromocriptine had any adverse effects on postnatal development. Weil (1986) compiled data on 86 patients (with 93 gestations) treated with bromocriptine during pregnancy to prevent visual complications caused by prolactinoma expansion. No significant effects of bromocriptine on the course of pregnancy, on delivery, or on the offspring were reported.

Pituitary Adenoma and Pregnancy

Gemzell and Wang (1979) reviewed the outcome of 217 pregnancies in 187 patients with pituitary adenomas. In patients with microadenomas, 94.5% of all pregnancies were uneventful. However, in patients with previously untreated macroprolactinomas, the complication rate during pregnancy was considerably higher; headaches and visual disturbances were reported in 25% of these cases. Griffith et al. (1979) reported on 137 prolactinoma patients. Of the 116 completed pregnancies in these patients, 8 were accompanied by visual disturbances and severe headaches were observed in 9 pregnancies. With the exception of craniotomies performed in two cases and bromocriptine re-institution in one, no further interventions were required. It should be mentioned that large tumors had been diagnosed in the two patients requiring surgery. From the data on the outcome of pregnancies in patients with comparable adenoma sizes, it can be deduced that complications are found predominantly in those patients who harbor an adenoma large enough to be documented by radiology and who have high prolactin levels before pregnancy. Almost all patients with pituitary prolactinomas and no evidence of extrasellar extension before pregnancy failed to show any signs of tumor enlargement during gestation. Therefore, the presence of microprolactinoma does not constitute a contraindication for ovulation induction, although close surveillance through monthly visual field determinations and clinical examinations of the patients throughout gestation is required.

Experimental data indicate that bromocriptine treatment not only decreases the secretory activity of pituitary lactotrophs, but also inhibits the reproductive mechanism of these cells, enabling a reduction in the volume of prolactinomas. Regression of prolactinoma size in response to bromocriptine therapy is now well-established. This effect can be expected in 40–80% of the patients with macroprolactinomas (Chiodini et al. 1981; Corenblum & Hanley, 1981). The initial and rapid effect (within days) is expressed in the amelioration of headaches and visual field defects. One can speculate that this primary effect is due to a decrease of peritumoral edema. The long-term (months) effect of bromocriptine demonstrates real regression in tumor size. However, bromocriptine does not permanently decrease the size of the tumors, and a rapid increase of the adenoma size and prolactin levels appears after discontinuing the drug (Thorner et al. 1981).

This antitumoral effect gives further support to the use of pharmacological therapy for pituitary tumors. In view of the disappointing results of pituitary surgery of macroprolactinomas, a trial of bromocriptine is usually warranted prior to surgery (Corenblum & Taylor, 1983; Barbieri & Ryan, 1983; Franks & Jacobs, 1983; Landolt, 1981).

In many cases, bromocriptine therapy alone will produce adequate anatomical and hormonal results.

In microprolactinomas, although the decrease in size is more difficult to assess and the results of transsphenoidal surgery are better, bromocriptine therapy is considered the first choice of therapy. This therapy can achieve the results of inducing ovulation and reducing prolactin levels without a significant risk of tumor expansion and with the preservation of all the other anterior pituitary functions.

The alternative to the conservative approach offered by bromocriptine therapy is surgical treatment. In cases of the failure of bromocriptine therapy, surgery is recommended both for micro- and macroprolactinomas (Barbieri & Ryan, 1983; Franks & Jacobs, 1983). In spite of enthusiasm for the transsphenoidal microsurgery technique, it must be recognized that the failure rate (recurrence or incomplete removal) in macroadenomas is 55% (Landolt, 1981; Schlechte et al. 1981).

Among these cases, the risk is greatest during pregnancy. Mortality in pituitary surgery is very low (0.4%). Complications such as diabetes insipidus (2%), early leak of cerebro-spinal fluid (CSF) (4.4%), and a late leak of CSF (2%) have been documented.

Serri et al. (1983), assessing long-term results of successful transsphenoidal adenomectomy in women with prolactinomas, concluded that late recurrences of hyperprolactinemia are high, ranging from 50% in microadenomas to 80% in macroadenomas. Our experience confirms these results (Berezin & Lunenfeld, 1983). However, if bromocriptine was initiated following surgery, no recurrence could be demonstrated during a long-term follow-up. Investigations on the natural history of microadenoma suggest that the tumors almost never progress to macroadenomas (March et al. 1981; Koppelman et al. 1984).

Furthermore, slow growth of prolactinomas and spontaneous remissions support the possibility of a conservative approach. The possibility of resuming bromocriptine therapy during pregnancy offers an additional alternative to the management of complications due to prolactinoma growth during gestation. We believe that treatment with bromocriptine as a sole therapy is satisfactory for the majority of patients with prolactinomas. The role of surgical treatment is becoming progressively reduced and should be confined to patients with extrasellar manifestations. If the pretreatment CT-scan shows suprasellar extension of a large adenoma, we advocate primary treatment with bromocriptine (for 2–6 weeks) followed by (transsphenoidal) surgery when the tumor size is reduced.

Side Effects

The main side effects of bromocriptine include orthostatic hypotension (usually asymptomatic), faintness, dizziness, nausea, and vomiting; collapse and a shock-like syndrome have also been described. It seems that puerperal women are less sensitive to side effects than are acromegalics and patients with Parkinson's disease. However, a gradual increase in the therapeutic dosage starting with 1.25 mg daily and the administration of the drug with food are recommended to reduce side effects and especially the first-dose phenomenon.

Other kinds of complications include mental disorders induced by treatment with bromocriptine and similar agents (Ferrari et al. 1976), even with low dosages. The spectrum of mental dysfunctions included delusional ideation, mania, and relapse of schizophrenia.

In patients developing side effects to any one of the available ergoline derivatives, a change to another compound of the same group may be beneficial.

OTHER PROLACTIN-INHIBITING AGENTS

The dopaminomimetic properties of ergot compounds have attracted much attention in recent years. When studied in sufficient detail, each ergot compound shows an individual profile of dopaminergic activities, thus providing ample opportunity for optimizing the pharmacodynamic properties of new drugs.

Several drugs, mostly ergoline derivatives like bromocriptine itself, have been studied as prolactin-lowering agents. The effect of some of these compounds is attributed to their activity as dopamine agonists. For others such as cyproheptadine, methysergide, and metergoline, the mechanism of action could be through a blockade of serotonin receptors, although this is still under debate.

Metergoline

The clavine derivative metergoline (Fig. 6-1), first developed as an antiserotonin agent, has a chemical structure resembling that of bromocriptine. In the last decade it has been observed that metergoline is also able to lower prolactin levels. A single intramuscular injection of metergoline significantly reduces prolactin levels in hyperprolactinemic women (Fig. 6-2), in lactating women, in regularly menstruating women, and in men. This drug most probably acts at the pituitary level via serotonin antagonism (Ferrari, 1976, 1980). In addition it has been shown that metergoline has a weak dopaminergic agonistic effect, especially when given in higher dosages.

Ferrari et al. (1980) studied the effect of metergoline in 41 hyperprolactinemic women. In this group, 35 women suffered from anovulation and, following treatment, 19 ovulated.

Lisuride

Lisuride hydrogen maleate (Fig. 6-1) was first demonstrated to possess antiserotoninergic activity (Votava & Lamplova, 1961), but later it was shown to have potent dopamine agonist properties (Horowski & Wachtel, 1976). This drug reduced prolactin response to TSH in normal males (Delitola et al. 1979). Treatment of hyperprolactinemia with this drug was effective in lowering plasma prolactin and in resuming ovulatory cycles (Bohnet et al. 1979). Table 6-3 shows the outcome of 540 pregnancies following lisuride treatment. Lisuride is usually administered twice daily in doses ranging from 50 – 200 μg. In the higher dosage range, signs of dopaminergic overstimulation such as drowsiness and nausea have been reported.

Pergolide

The ergot derivative pergolide mesilate (Fig. 6-1) seems to possess very potent prolactin-inhibiting properties and a long duration of action. A single dose of 100 to 400 μg lowers prolactin levels for more than 24 hours (Lemberger & Crabtree, 1979).

TABLE 6-3. Pregnancies in hyperprolactinamic Women after Treatment with Dopergin®
(Lisuride)

Outcome of Pregnancies		No. of Cases
Birth	normal birth	373
	cesarean section	52
	premature delivery	26
	vacuum ectraction	16
	forceps	4
	stillbirth	2
	multiple birth	5
		478
Abortion	spontaneous abortion	31
	missed abortion	14
	induced abortion	4
	fetal death at 20 weeks	2
	incomplete abortion	3
	extrauterine pregnancy	6
	hydatidiform mole	2
		62
Total Pregnancies		540

Clinical trials by Callaghan et al. (1981) and Franks et al. (1981) confirmed the efficacy of this drug in decreasing prolactin hypersecretion and the resumption of ovulatory cycles. Similar results were reported by Blackwell et al. (1983).

Reduction of macroadenomas and microadenomas using pergolide treatment was described by Kleinberg et al. (1983).

Crosignani et al. (1982) compared the effect of three ergot derivatives, bromocriptine, metergoline, and lisuride, in 191 cases of hyperprolactinemia of various origin. Of 115 cases treated by bromocriptine, ovulation was achieved in 64 and pregnancy in 44 (38%). In 23 cases treated with lisuride, an ovulation rate of 25% and a pregnancy rate of 14% were achieved. Of the 82 patients treated by metergoline, 42 ovulated and 9 (11%) became pregnant. These results indicate the superiority of bromocriptine in terms of pregnancy rate. Other multi-center studies compared the efficacy of bromocriptine and pergolide in hyperprolactinemia (Swyer et al. 1978). The patients' responses to both drugs were similar in decreasing prolactin hypersecretion, resolution of amenorrhea, galactorrhea, and diminution of adenoma size. The side effects were similar, as well.

It seems that cases refractory to one of the ergoline derivatives might benefit from treatment with others of the same pharmacological group.

It is at present quite clear that bromocryptine and other ergoline derivatives should be regarded as ovulation-inducing drugs with great potential. In the case of therapeutic failures, treatment with clomiphene/hCG or hMG/hCG or FSH/hCG or pulsatile GnRH application are highly effective.

The clinical experience gleaned from the application of ergoline derivatives shows without any doubt that these drugs are an important addition to the armamentarium available for the treatment of infertility in hyperprolactinemic anovulatory patients.

7. HUMAN GONADOTROPHINS

HISTORICAL BACKGROUND

The first steps towards the clinical use of gonadotrophins were actually taken in the mid-twenties when Zondek and Smith independently but almost simultaneously discovered that gonadal function was controlled by the pituitary gland.

Zondek (1926a, 1926b) demonstrated that implantation of anterior pituitary caused a rapid development of sexual organs in immature animals. At approximately the same time, Smith and his group showed that hypophysectomy resulted in a failure of sexual maturation in immature animals and in a rapid regression of sexual characteristics in adult animals (Smith, 1926; Smith & Engle, 1927).

During the 1930s and 1940s, gonadotrophin extracts from different animal materials were prepared and applied for the stimulation of ovarian function in humans. It has been quickly realized, however, that these preparations were of very limited clinical value because nonprimate gonadotrophins produced in the human a rapid immunological response neutralizing their therapeutic effect (Leethem & Rakoff, 1948). This focused scientific and technological efforts on the extraction and purification of gonadotropins from human sources. Intensive research in this area was simultaneously carried out in Italy, England, Scotland, Switzerland, and Sweden. In the late 1950s and early 1960s, these efforts were crowned by success. Gemzell and his co-workers reported the first successful induction of ovulation using human pituitary gonadotrophin in 1958 and the first pregnancy in 1960 (Gemzell et al. 1958, 1960). Approximately at the same time, Bettendorf succeeded in extracting a potent gonadotrophic agent from human pituitaries and reported on first clinical experience with its use (Bettendorf et al. 1961). Lunenfeld and his group, working with urinary extracts of human menopausal gonadotrophin (hMG), achieved ovulations and pregnancies in anovulatory women. Their results were reported at various scientific and medical meetings, beginning in 1959 and later published in 1963 (Lunenfeld, 1963), and remained the standard for ovulation induction till today.

Large-scale clinical studies were then undertaken in numerous centers throughout the world and their results reported in the literature. Of particular significance were the reports of Bettendorf (1966) and Gemzell (1973), who were able to induce ovulation and pregnancy in hypophysectomized women.

The introduction of rapid and reliable hormonal assays and later the availability of ultrasound scanners enabling visualization and measurement of ovarian follicles made monitoring of gonadotrophin therapy accurate and objective and improved the results of treatment.

In the 1980s, the large-scale in vitro fertilization (IVF) programs used the principles developed for and the experience gained from induction of ovulation in infertile patients and added new important insights to the understanding of the mechanism of ovarian stimulation by gonadotropins.

Table 7-1 describes shortly the most important milestones of the long and tedious way which led from the discovery of the gonadotrophic principle to in vitro fertilization.

The induction of ovulation with human gonadotropins has been an integral part of the routine work of many fertility clinics for more than 30 years. During that time numerous reports describing all aspects of gonadotrophin therapy in great detail have been published (Thompson & Hansen, 1970; Insler & Lunenfeld, 1974; Lunenfeld & Insler, 1978; Brown, 1986).

TABLE 7-1. Milestones in the Development of Gonadotrophin Therapy

1920s and 1930s	* Discovery of the gonadotrophic principle controlling ovarian function
1930–1940	* Further insights into the physiology of Hypothalamic-Pituitary-Ovarian axis
	* Extraction of gonadotrophins from animal sources and from human pregnancy urine
1950	* Extraction of gonadotropins from human pituitaries and post-menopausal urine
1960s	* Large-scale extraction and purification processes for human gonadotropins
	* Clinical studies of ovulation induction using hPG and hMG
	* Introduction of quick and reliable hormone assays for monitoring of therapy
1970s	* Large-scale clinical use of gonadotrophins in infertile patients
	* Introduction of sonography for monitoring ovulation-inducing therapy
1980s	* Controlled superovulation (hyperstimulation) therapy used in IVF/ET programs

Human urinary follicle-stimulating hormone (FSH) as alternative to hMG has become commercially available in the late eighties. It offers theoretical advantages over hMG when used for induction of ovulation in patients with polycystic ovarian disease (PCOD). Because PCOD is characterized by abnormally elevated serum LH levels, the use of the purified FSH is attractive, since it contains virtually no LH. During the last few years FSH is being used either in combination with hMG or as an alternative to hMG in many ovulation inducing protocols or IVF programs. Although many reports describing and comparing the clinical characteristics of ovulation induction with hMG and FSH have appeared in the literature it is still equivocal whether "pure" FSH it is significantly more effective than hMG.

The population size of women between 19–34 in the developed world in 1990 has been above 130 million, and if we assume that at least 8 % are infertile, then the pool of the infertile population would be above 10 million with about 700,000 new patients entering this pool every year between 1990 and 1995 (Lunenfeld, 1990).

The future of infertility therapy clearly relies on the capacity to produce pharmaceutical grade gonadotrophins in sufficient quantities to meet this ever increasing world-wide demand. With recombinant DNA technology and highly refined cell culture techniques recombinant DNA gonadotrophins are being prepared. What would currently require 200 million litres of urine will ultimately be produced by genetically engineered cells in chemical defined culture medium comprising only a small fraction of that volume. The initial challenge involved construction of appropriate vectors for inserting alpha and beta subunit DNA into well-characterized and stable cells. Unlike Insulin and growth hormone, the gonadotropins are glycosylated heterodimeric peptides. The complex sugars are important for proper folding of the polypeptide backbone. The sites and extent of glycosylation determine tertiary structure, length of time of degradation, the regions of the molecule exposed to target cell receptors, and exposure of the molecule to mechanisms that regulate metabolism in vivo. Whereas bacteria efficiently produce nonglycosylated peptides such as Insulin, and yeast has been cloned for the production of certain vaccine, prokaryotic cells are incapable of correctly glycosylating the peptide subunits to produce biologically active gonadotropins. Since the Chinese hamster ovary cells are known to be suitable host cells for the production of glycosylated recombinant proteins, such cell lines were chosen for the expression of recombinant human FSH. To obtain this goal, cloned human FSH genes were inserted in an expression vector and transferred to the Chinese hamster ovary cell line. Specific cell clones have now been selected for large-scale production of recombinant FSH. The resultant preparations are very pure and have a biological potency > 10,000 IU/mg. It is our hope that in the not too distant future recombinant DNA technology will provide an almost unlimited supply of human gonadotropins.

CHEMISTRY CLEARANCE AND PHYSIOLOGY

During the last 30 years, the major elements of the mechanism of action, control, and regulation of secretion of gonadotropins has been elucidated, and more recently, their structure has been determined.

Gonadotropins have been found to be glycoproteins with molecular weights around 30,000 daltons and containing about 20% carbohydrates. The carbohydrate moieties in their molecules are fucose, mannose, galactose, acetylglucosamine and N-acetylneuroaminic acid (Butt & Kennedy, 1971). The sialic acid content varies widely among the glycoprotein hormones, from 20 residues in hCG and 5 in FSH to only one or two in hLH. These differences are largely responsible for the variations in the isoelectric points of gonadotropins.

The carbohydrate moieties are complex. They may be branched or straight chains and they contain sialic acid as an important constituent, particularly at the end of the chains.

Different sialic acid content accounts for differences in the molecular weight of the hormones isolated from various sources and in differences in biological activity determined in in vivo assays. The higher the sialic acid content, the longer the biological half-life. Thus, the increased amount of carbohydrate in hCG is responsible for its significantly longer half-life than that of LH or FSH. For this reason desialized preparations of hLH, hCG, and hFSH show considerably reduced biological activity in vivo but retain activity in specific in vitro biological assays employing membrane receptors or isolated target cells.

The gonadotropic hormones consist of two hydrophobic noncovalently associated alpha and beta subunits. The pure subunits are practically without biological activity, but the activity is regenerated by allowing the two subunits to recombine. All the gonadotropins as well as thyroid-stimulating hormone (TSH) share a common alpha subunit of 92 amino acid residues in the same sequence with 5 disulfide bonds as well as 2 carbohydrate moieties. The beta subunits (of FSH, LH, and hCG) are unique to each hormone and confer their biologic specificity. They have amino acid chains of variable lengths (116–147 amino acid residues) and contain six disulfide bonds.

Methodologies which have allowed the analysis of the genes and gene products have shown that the two subunits of the gonadotropic hormones are translated from separate messenger RNAs (Fiddes & Goodman, 1979) and both are synthesized as precursors. The nascent polypeptide alpha and beta subunits are then glycosylated and finally the alpha and beta subunits then combine noncovalently in a two-step reaction to form the biologically active glycoproteins (Hussa, 1980).

The information regarding metabolism of gonadotropic hormones is scarce. It has been shown that purified preparations of hFSH, hLH, and hCG injected intravenously into humans had serum half-lives (as determined by bioassays) of 180-240 minutes, 42-60 minutes, and 6-8 hours respectively. The half-life of the alpha and beta subunit of LH was found to be only 16 minutes. The higher carbohydrate content of hCG (10%) is responsible for its significantly longer half-life than hFSH (5%) and hLH (2%).

The mean metabolic clearance rate (MCR) of hFSH in women has been determined to be 14 ml/min. and has not been determined in men. The MCR of hLH is 25-30 ml/min. in women, regardless of ovulatory state, and is almost 50% higher in normal men. The disappearance curves for both hormones are multi-exponential, indicating a distribution of these hormones in more than three mathematical compartments. In premenopausal women, daily production rates of hLH are 500-1,000 IU with a marked preovulatory rise, whereas production rates in postmenopausal women are 3,000 to 4,000 IU per day. These values indicate that the pituitary content of hLH (and probably of hFSH) is turned over once or twice daily and that rapid biosynthesis of gonadotropins must be necessary to maintain the normal levels of pituitary storage and secretion.

Only 3-10% of the daily production of FSH and LH is excreted in the urine in a biologically active form, but reflects the rate of gonadotropin secretion in physiologic and pathologic conditions. The recovery of exogenous gonadotropins in the urine of normal and infertile subjects is 10-20% of the administered hormone. Urinary excretion of gonadotropins accounts for only 5% of the MCR. The MCR of hMG in hypogonadotropic subjects is 0.4-1.7 ml/min.

THE RATIONALE AND THE AIMS OF GONADOTROPHIN THERAPY

The rationale of gonadotropin treatment is to provide gonadotropin levels of magnitude and timing similar to those observed in a normal ovulatory cycle and, consequently, to evoke recruitment of a follicular cohort, selection and full maturation of at least one dominant follicle, ovulation, and sustained corpus luteum function.

Unfortunately, this goal has never been fully achieved. The FSH and LH levels and their ratios during gonadotropin-stimulated cycles are quite different from normal (Wu, 1977; Healy & Burger, 1982). Estrogen levels and their daily rate of ascent as well as progesterone values differ from those observed in spontaneous cycles (Insler & Potashnik, 1983). The follicular fluid levels of estradiol and progesterone are lower and the level of inhibin is higher in preovulatory gonadotropin-stimulated cycles than in the dominant follicle of the natural cycle (Seegar-Jones et al. 1985).

Moreover, the pregnancy rate in gonadotropin-induced cycles with steroid profiles closely resembling those found in spontaneous ovulations is dismally low (Insler & Lunenfeld, 1977). Thus, the theoretical rationale of gonadotropin therapy must be subordinated to its clinical aim which is: to obtain ovulation and pregnancy in all suitable cases while avoiding hyperstimulation.

Large-scale clinical experience indicates that this goal can be practically achieved. The unequivocal proof of the clinical efficiency of gonadotropin therapy is the thousands of babies born following gonadotropin-induced ovulations and conceptions.

SELECTION OF PATIENTS

Gonadotrophin treatment is primarily a substitution therapy and as such should be applied in patients lacking appropriate gonadotropin stimulation but having target organs (gonads) capable of normal response.

In daily practice, however, gonadotropins are also used in other groups of patients.

In 1968, Insler et al. proposed a simple treatment-oriented classification of patients selected for gonadotrophin therapy. This classification has been modified and adopted by the WHO Scientific Group (World Health Organization, Technical Report Series, 1976) and is used in many centers until the present day.

According to this classification (see Fig. 3-1) gonadotropin treatment is applied in two main groups of women:

Group I:
Hypothalamic-Pituitary Failure – amenorrheic women with no evidence of endogenous estrogen production, with nonelevated prolactin levels, with normal or low FSH levels and no detectable space-occupying lesion in the hypothalamic-pituitary region.

Group II:
Hypothalamic-Pituitary Dysfunction – women with a variety of menstrual cycle disturbances including amenorrhea with evidence of endogenous estrogen production and normal levels of prolactin and FSH. It seems that a significant number of patients of Group II, particularly those showing signs of hyperandrogenism, may actually suffer from polycystic ovarian disease (PCOD) (Hull, 1989; Insler & Lunenfeld, 1990; Insler & Lunenfeld, 1991).

In Group II gonadotropins are usually applied after other types of ovulation-inducing therapy have failed.

It is theoretically plausible and clinically proven that the results of gonadotropin treatment are significantly better in Group I as compared to Group II (Lunenfeld et al. 1981). Amenorrheic women of Group I, however, represent only a small and ever-diminishing proportion of the infertility clinic population (Bettendorf et al. 1981a).

In recent years another, steadily growing in numbers, group of patients is being treated with human gonadotropins: women being subjected to in vitro fertilization.

Obviously, these patients differ from both Group I and Group II in having completely normal hormonal levels and competent hypothalamic-pituitary-ovarian feedback mechanisms.

The general principles of gonadotropin therapy applied to the above-mentioned three groups of patients are similar, but the intensity of stimulation, course of treatment, and hormonal patterns differ significantly.

It may thus be summarized that, at present, three modes of gonadotrophin treatment are used:

Substitution therapy	– applied in patients of Group I
Stimulation therapy	– given to patients of Group II
Controlled-Hyperstimulation therapy	– used in IVF programs

PRINCIPLES OF GONADOTROPHIN THERAPY

The basic principles of gonadotropin therapy were proposed by Insler & Lunenfeld (1974, 1977) following observation of the course of treatment in several hundreds of patients. Ovarian response can be elicited only when a certain dose of FSH-like material has been applied. This amount of gonadotropins is called the EFFECTIVE DAILY DOSE. Administration of gonadotropins at levels significantly below the effective daily dose does not evoke any measurable effect even when prolonged therapy is used.

Following the application of the effective daily dose of gonadotropins, a number of ovarian follicles is stimulated to begin its growth and maturation. This period of gonadotropin therapy is called the LATENT PHASE. Since at this stage of follicular development appreciable amounts of estrogen are not yet secreted, and since the size of the follicles is too small to be precisely measured by ultrasound the latent phase of therapy is clinically "mute". The latent phase begins with the application of the effective daily dose of gonadotropins and ends with the appearance of measurable ovarian response, i.e. rising estrogen levels and increasing follicular diameter.

The second part of gonadotropin therapy, called the ACTIVE PHASE, lasts from the initial estrogen rise until ovulation induction. It is characterized by an exponential rise of estrogen levels and a steady growth of follicular diameter (Fig. 7–1).

The duration of the latent phase is 3 to 7 days and is significantly longer in patients of Group I than in women of Group II. The length of the active phase is 4 to 6 days and is similar in all patients.

The above principles, based on clinical observation and the thorough analysis of patients' responses, received a powerful theoretical support from the experimental work of Hodgen and his group on primates (Goodman et al. 1977; Hodgen, 1982; Hodgen et al. 1983). The introduction of sonography for the monitoring of follicular size and the IVF programs allowing for direct laparoscopic observation of the size and appearance of ovarian follicles concomitant with the appreciation of the maturity of ova lend further support to the empirically developed principles of gonadotropin therapy.

According to Hodgen's work in primates, the sequence of events leading to ovulation is as follows:

* RECRUITMENT of a follicular cohort – is brought about by a slight but significant FSH rise observed during the preceding late luteal phase. This process is completed by the 3rd cycle day.

* SELECTION of the dominant follicle – is a process by which one follicle of the cohort is endowed with the ability to mature earlier and/or quicker than all others. The exact mechanism of the selection process is not yet known. Our own theory is

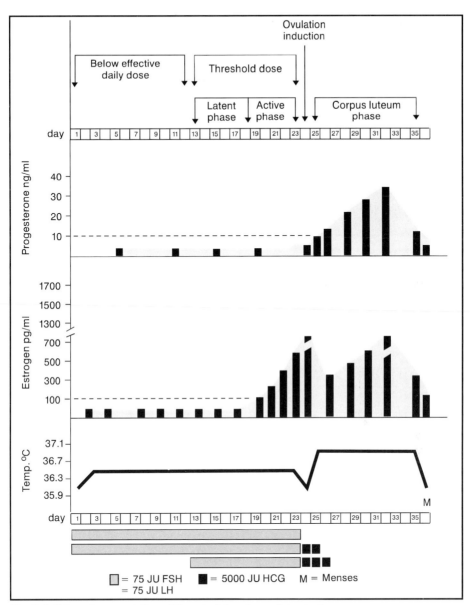

Fig. 7-1. Schematic presentation of the principles of gonadotropin therapy.

that the "assignment" of the follicle to be selected as the dominant one in the next cycle is brought about by the rescuing action of the midcycle FSH peak in the previous cycle. The process of selection of the dominant follicle is completed by the 7th cycle day.

* DOMINANCE - is that part of the cycle when all the events such as the exponential rise of estrogen, negative feedback action upon the hypothalamus, modulation of pituitary secretion of gonadotropins, reduction of FSH-secretion by inhibin, and

positive feedback evoking the midcycle LH-surge are subordinated to the developmental rhythm of the dominant follicle. This controlling action of the dominant follicle lasts from the 8th cycle day until ovulation and also persists during the corpus luteum phase (Fig. 7-2).

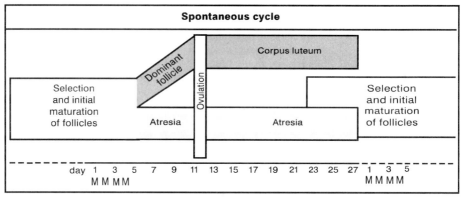

Fig. 7-2. Schematic presentation of the sequence of events during spontaneous ovulatory cycle. (From: V. Insler, Gonadotropin therapy – new trends and insights, Int. J. Fertil. 1988)

The latent phase of gonadotrophin therapy represents a "telescoped in" version of the recruitment and selection phase of the spontaneous cycle. The active phase of therapy corresponds to the period of dominance (Fig. 7-3).

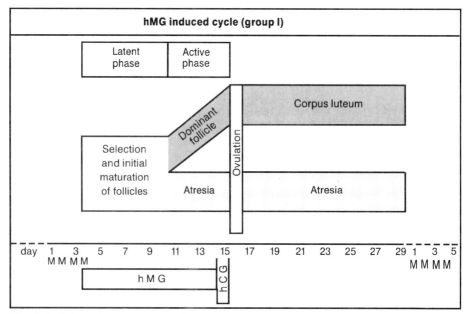

Fig. 7-3. Schematic presentation of the sequence of events during hMG-induced cycle in a hypopituitary hypogonadotrophic patient (Group I).
(From: V. Insler, Gonadotrophin therapy – new trends and insights, Int. J. Fertil. 1988)

The question of differences of response observed in patients of Group I as compared to those of Group II must now be briefly addressed. It is well known that in patients of Group II the effective daily dose is smaller, the latent phase is shorter, and the response to treatment is less uniform (Insler & Lunenfeld, 1977). It seems that

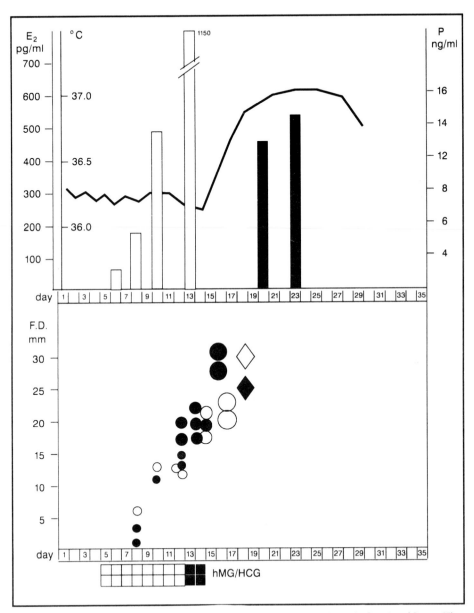

Fig. 7-4. Gonadotrophin therapy in a patient with hypothalamic-pituitary dysfunction (Group II).
E-2 = serum estradiol
P   = plasma progesterone
FD   = follicular diameter – in the left ovary (black circles), right ovary (empty circles), black and white rhomboides represent corpora lutea in respective ovaries

these differences in response to stimulation with exogenous gonadotropins may be explained by the state of the ovary at the beginning of treatment.

In women of Group I, at the initiation of each treatment course, the ovaries are at a quiescent state with almost all follicles at a low stage of development. The pharmacological dose of gonadotropins applied acts on a relatively uniform substrate. Not so in patients of Group II. In this group, endogenous gonadotropins may cause a certain follicular development before or between treatments. Gonadotropin therapy is thus applied to an ovary containing already scores of follicles at various stages of development, provoking further growth of some of them, recruitment of additional ones, and atresia of others. No wonder that the response to treatment is less uniform and more prone to hyperstimulation (Fig. 7-4).

Gonadotropin therapy poses several interesting theoretical problems.

The exact size of the follicular cohort recruited in each cycle in the human is not known. It is thus impossible to know whether gonadotropin therapy, using unphysiological doses, provokes initial development of a larger cohort. Whatever the size of the initial cohort recruited, it seems that, during the course of gonadotropin therapy, additional follicles are stimulated and undergo partial or full maturation and others are rescued from atresia by the sustained high level of FSH. This process results in the development of several dominant follicles that reach full maturity hours or maybe even days apart from each other.

As indicated by the very low efficiency of single dose or "trigger" schemes of therapy, to ensure follicular maturation during gonadotropin therapy, relatively high FSH levels must be sustained throughout the treatment.

It is of interest to note that despite the rather high levels of estrogen occurring relatively early in treatment, premature LH-surges are rather rare (Garcia et al. 1983). This is true in patients with hypothalamic-pituitary failure, but in patients with hypothalamic-pituitary dysfunction they may occur in 25% of all treatment cycles (Fleming et al. 1988). According to studies in primates (Schenken & Hodgen, 1983, Sopelak & Hodgen, 1984), the hyperstimulated ovary may secrete a Gonadotropin Surge Inhibiting Factor (different from inhibin) which blocks the LH-surge triggered by the rising estrogen levels.

When using human gonadotropins to induce ovulation, one has to accept the fact that some features of spontaneous ovulatory cycle can not be reproduced in gonadotropin-induced cycles. These features are:
* Premenstrual recruitment and initial selection of follicles
* Feedback control of gonadotropin levels
* Balanced effect of intraovarian sex steroids
* Full maturation of one follicle only
* Exact synchronization of structural, functional, and hormonal events throughout the entire genital system.

Recently it has been demonstrated that somatomedin-C in nanomolar concentrations enhances FSH capacity to induce progesterone production by cultured rat granulosa cells (Adashi et al. 1985). Furthermore, growth factors have been shown to modulate the effects of FSH in the differentiation process of granulosa cells (Davoren & Hsueh, 1986). This indicates that growth hormone (GH) is capable of stimulating various growth factors that enhance FSH action on granulosa cells. Preliminary clinical experiments demonstrated that combined growth hormone/gonadotropin therapy significantly increased the ovarian response to exogenous gonadotropins in patients with pituitary insufficiency (including GH deficiency) and in women with hyposensitive ovaries (Homburg et al. 1988, Blumenfeld + Lunenfeld 1989).

TREATMENT SCHEMES

A whole array of treatment schemes for gonadotropin therapy have been proposed and employed over the years. There are, however, only three essentially different types of therapy:

*   fixed dose regimes
**   individually adjusted schemes
***   combined therapy

In the fixed dose regimes, a certain amount of hMG (or HPG) is administered on predetermined cycle days, followed by hCG given one or more days after the last injection of hMG/FSH (HPG). Although the dosages of gonadotropins and the days on which it was administered differed in various reports (Crooke, 1970; Marshall & Jacobson, 1970; Butler, 1970), the general principle was identical. By using a fixed dose in each cycle, the patient's gonadotropin requirement (i.e. the effective daily dose) could be met only by successively increasing the dose in consecutive cycles.

The individually adjusted treatment scheme (Rabau et al. 1971) allows for successive increments of the gonadotropin dose according to the patient's response during the same cycle. It thus comprises the tests courses with the treatment course in one cycle, thus significantly increasing the efficiency of treatment (mean number of treatment courses per pregnancy). In some particularly sensitive cases, the individually adjusted treatment may avoid hyperstimulation, which would have been brought about by using the fixed dose schedule.

The problem of the size of the initial dose of hMG/FSH and of its increments as well as the ideal estrogen level to be arrived at before application of hCG is still a matter of discussion. We usually start with 2 ampules of hMG/FSH per day in patients of Group I and with 1 ampule in women belonging to Group II. The successive dose increments are usually by one ampule each, and hCG is administered when urinary estrogen reaches a level of 75 to 200 µg/24h or plasma estradiol attains a level of 300 to 900 pg/ml (see Fig. 7-1).

In PCOD patients a low-dose with stepwise increase treatment scheme has been proposed (Seibel et al. 1984; Sagle et al. 1991; Shoham et al. 1991) According to this protocol FSH (or hMG) is started at 75 IU daily and increased by half of this amount after 7 or 14 days if no adequate response has been achieved, as evidenced by sonographic or hormonal parameters.

It is interesting to note that, with the advent of IVF programs, the whole cycle of trial and error regarding the most efficient and safe treatment schemes of hMG/FSH was repeated. Different groups proposed fixed dose schedules not much different from those which were tried and discarded years ago. Recently, however, more and more groups seem to adopt the individually adjusted treatment scheme, using some modifications suitable for the special purposes of an IVF program (Quigley, 1985; Lopata et al. 1986).

For the sake of completeness, one additional mode of ovulation-induction using human gonadotropins should be mentioned here. In 1983, Kemmann et al. described their initial experience with a portable infusion pump delivering subdermally a constant amount of hMG/FSH over a period of 18 hours per day. The authors claimed that with this method of delivery a better response was obtained than with the standard i.m. injection of hMG/FSH.

Combined Treatment

In the past, most IVF programs used a combination of clomiphene citrate and hMG/FSH to stimulate a large enough crop of follicles ready for ovum pick-up. The claim was that this combination produced better, or at least more uniform, ovum maturation than hMG/FSH alone. Proof for this claim has, however, not been established. Moreover, this mode of treatment is being abandoned because of the long half-life of clomiphene citrate and the high incidence of untimely LH-surges.

It is well known that patients of Group I respond better to gonadotropin therapy than women of Group II. The efficiency of treatment (mean number of treatment courses per pregnancy) and the pregnancy rate are significantly better in the former group as compared to the latter (Lunenfeld et al. 1981).

Some of the reasons for this discrepancy are obvious.

Firstly, patients of Group II receive gonadotropin therapy only after they have failed to conceive when treated with other ovulation-inducing drugs. Second, the frequency of additional disturbances possibly affecting fertility, such as endometriosis, tubal factor, and polycystic ovaries, are much more frequent in Group II.

There are, however, differences in response to stimulation between patients of Group I and those of Group II which seem to be inherent to the functional characteristics of the hypothalamic-pituitary-ovarian axis (see Section: Principles of gonadotropin therapy). In other words, with regard to gonadotropin therapy, the presence of a functioning pituitary gland may be a disadvantage rather than an asset.

To overcome the possible interference of untimely and/or unbalanced endogenous gonadotropin secretion, combined therapy using agents suppressing hypothalamic-pituitary function together with hMG or a purified FSH preparation was recommended.

Ben-Nun and Lunenfeld (1984) generated pharmacological (drug-induced) hyperprolactinemia, causing a significant reduction of secretion and/or release of endogenous gonadotropins, and then stimulated the ovaries by exogenous hMG/FSH. They claimed that, with this type of combined treatment, ovulations and pregnancies could be obtained in several patients of Group II who previously failed to conceive when treated with hMG/hCG alone.

Laboratory synthesis of potent and/or long-acting analogs of gonadotropin-releasing hormone (GnRH) makes it possible to efficiently reduce (down-regulate) the production and release of pituitary gonadotropins (Borgman et al. 1982; Crawley et al. 1982; Meldrum et al. 1982; Yen, 1983).

Treatment schemes combining pituitary suppression by GnRH analogs with ovarian stimulation by exogenous gonadotropins seemed therefore particularly attractive.

Bettendorf et al. (1981b) reported on the preliminary results of this treatment module. They used buserelin nasal spray to suppress pituitary function and hMG/FSH/hCG to induce ovulation. However, in this trial the extent of pituitary down-regulation was ascertained by assays of basal levels of FSH and LH only, and not by dynamic tests. Moreover, in some cases the GnRH analog was discontinued before the application of gonadotropins.

TABLE 7-2. Comparison of Treatment and Response Parameters in combined GnRH Agonist/hMG/hCG Therapy and hMG/hCG Treatment

Parameter	GnRH Agonist + Gonadotrophins		Gonadotrophins alone	
	Mean	Range	Mean	Range
Duration of treatment (days)	16.6	3 – 28	11.1	5 – 20
Total hMG dose (amps.)	26.4	5 – 48	16.5	5 – 34
Effective daily dose (amps.)	1.7	1 – 3.5	1.7	1 – 3.0
Latent phase (days)	6.2	3 – 9	5.9	3 – 9
Active phase (days)	6.8	3 – 9	5.1	3 – 7

Recently, combined GnRH analog/gonadotrophin therapy is being re-tried by several different groups (Fleming et al. 1988; Hedon, 1988; Shadmi et al. 1987; Bettendorf et al. 1988; Lunenfeld et al. 1988). Our own experience with this type of treatment seems to be quite interesting (Insler et al. 1988). Pretreatment with GnRH agonists reduces significantly the FSH levels within 14–21 days. The reduction of LH levels is also apparent but is significant only in cases in which the basic levels were relatively high. In the majority of cases treated with either daily doses of Decapeptyl or with monthly injections of Decapeptyl CR (Ferring, West Germany) or with nasal spray applications of Buserelin (Hoechst, West Germany), the levels of plasma estradiol and the pituitary response to estradiol benzoate stimulation were also significantly reduced. Ovarian stimulation by gonadotrophins, when applied after down-regulation of the axis was achieved by GnRH agonist, required a higher hMG/FSH dose and a longer therapy and produced more follicles than the treatment by gonadotrophins alone (Table 7-2). However, these follicles were probably smaller and less competent, as indicated by the levels of E2, which were not significantly different in combined GnRH agonist/gonadotrophin as compared to gonadotrophin alone therapy (Fig. 7-5).

Figure 7-6 shows a course of combined GnRH analog/gonadotrophin therapy in a patient of Group II who was previously treated with repeated courses of clomiphene citrate and of hMG/FSH/hCG but failed to ovulate and/or conceive.

The full potential of the combined pituitary suppression/ovarian stimulation therapy can not yet be accurately assessed. To enable such an assessment, extensive and detailed information regarding the indications, the precise dosage and timing, and the best monitoring parameters will have to be generated and critically analyzed.

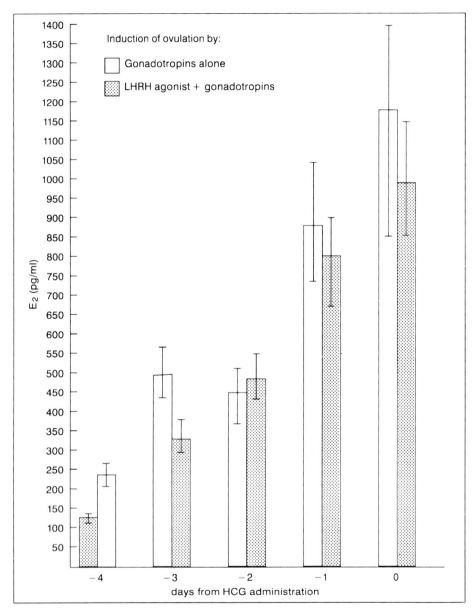

Fig. 7–5. Estradiol (E₂) levels in patients treated with gonadotrophins alone and in women receiving combined hMG/hCG/GnRH analog therapy.

MONITORING OF THERAPY

Proper monitoring is crucial for the results of gonadotrophin therapy, i.e. for achieving a high rate of conceptions while avoiding hyperstimulation and reducing the incidence of multiple pregnancy to an acceptable minimum. Monitoring of the ovarian response to stimulation has four objectives:

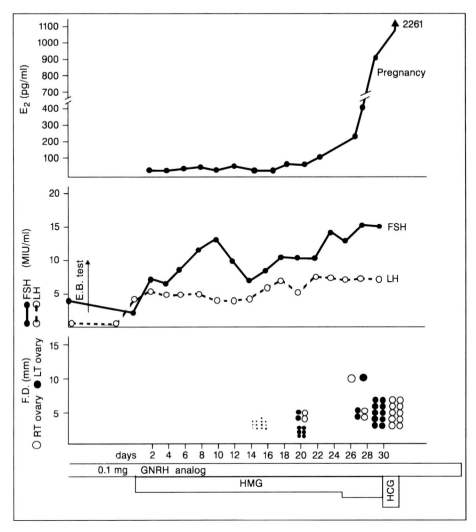

Fig. 7-6. Combined GnRH analog/gonadotrophin therapy in a patient with hypothalamic-pituitary dysfunction (Group II).
FD = sonographic measurements of follicular diameter

1. to determine the size of the effective (threshold) daily dose of hMG/FSH
2. to determine the duration of hMG/FSH administration
3. to determine the suitability, size, and timing of administration of the ovulatory dosage of hCG
4. to determine the occurrence and time of ovulation and to evaluate the corpus luteum function.

Three different types of parameters are used in the monitoring of gonadotrophin therapy:
*   clinical   ** hormonal   *** ultrasonic

Clinical parameters include vaginal examination, basal body temperature (BBT) records, and cervical mucus evaluation expressed as a semiquantitative cervical score (Insler et al. 1970; Insler et al. 1972); hormonal assays required for monitoring gonadotropin treatment consist of estrogen and progesterone estimations; the ultrasonic examinations are aimed at determining the number and size of ovarian follicles and, if possible, also at observing their postovulatory transformation into corpora lutea (Hackeloer, 1984; Cabau & Besis, 1981; Ritchie, 1985).

The latent phase of gonadotropin therapy is "mute" to monitoring. At that time neither the clinical nor the hormonal or ultrasonic parameters can give an objective measure of the ovarian response to stimulation. The role of monitoring at this stage is to establish the size of the effective daily dose of hMG/FSH. This is done empirically by successively increasing the daily dose of hMG/FSH by one ampule every 5–7 days until a distinct ovarian response begins as indicated by the initiation of steroidogenesis and by ultrasonically measurable follicular growth.

The main monitoring effort is centered at the active phase of treatment. The number of follicles developing and their growth rhythm must be established, and the time when at least one follicle is ready to receive the ovulatory LH stimulus must be determined as accurately as possible.

The lessons learned from in vitro fertilization indicate that, in order to carry out this complicated task, it is best to use all three monitoring parameters: clinical, hormonal, and ultrasonic. The number and diameter of follicles determined by ultrasound and the pattern of ascent of estrogen levels provide a good indication of the extent of follicular maturation. The clinical parameters (cervical score), in addition to being an indirect indicator of estrogen levels, reflect the functional state of the genital tract with regard to sperm transport.

It has been repeatedly shown that both plasma 17-beta-estradiol as well as urinary total estrogen may be used for monitoring of gonadotropin therapy with equal efficiency (Brown, 1986; Insler & Potashnik, 1983; Lequin et al. 1986).

A steady exponential rise of urinary or plasma estrogen is usually observed during the active phase of gonadotropin therapy. The ideal daily ascent rate is considered to be in the range of 40–100%. A slower ascent may reflect a suboptimal response and a steeper daily increase is a warning sign of an exaggerated response, possibly heralding hyperstimulation.

For many years, the dominant follicle was considered to be the main source of estrogen, the contribution of smaller follicles being regarded as marginal. In vitro fertilization and ultrasound proved that this is true in monofollicular cycles only. In cycles with multifollicular development, peripheral estrogen levels reflect the sum total of steroidogenic activity of several leading follicles as well as of a number of "runner-up" follicles. Nitschke-Dabelstein et al. (1981) showed that an excellent correlation between the 17-beta-estradiol levels and the number and size of follicles observed on ultrasound could be found in monofollicular but not in multifollicular cycles. On the other hand, the follicular size as measured by ultrasound is inadequate as a sole parameter of follicular maturation, the functional integrity of the follicle being probably better expressed by its steroidogenic activity.

This is the main reason for combining hormonal and sonographic parameters in monitoring gonadotropin therapy. A steady daily rise of estrogen levels concomitant with a constant growth of follicular diameter on ultrasound are the best indicators of successful ovarian stimulation as well as reasonably good predictors of hyperstimulation.

Practically monitoring of gonadotrophin treatment is carried out as follows (Figs. 7-1 and 7-4):

Patients are instructed to keep daily body temperature (BBT) records. Treatment is started between the 3rd and 5th day of spontaneous or induced bleeding. If combined GnRH analog/gonadotrophin therapy is applied, the treatment is started when a complete pituitary-ovarian down-regulation has been achieved. The initial hMG/FSH dose is usually 1 ampule per day in patients of Group II. In women of Group I and in patients receiving the combined therapy, treatment is usually started with 2 ampules per day. If the patient received gonadotropin therapy in the past, treatment is usually started at the level of the effective daily dose (EDD) of the previous course. Prior to initiation of every course of treatment, an ultrasonic scan of the pelvic region is performed in order to rule out the presence of abnormal follicular structures or cysts. Since such structures may interfere with ovarian response to stimulation, they should be punctured or the treatment should be delayed until their spontaneous disappearance.

Patients are examined every 1 to 3 days. This examination includes palpation of the ovaries, estimation of cervical score, postcoital tests when indicated, and a short interview with the patient regarding her general well-being. The dose of gonadotropins is adjusted according to the patient's response as indicated by estrogens, ultrasonography, and clinical findings.

If estrogens are low and not rising, the initial dose of gonadotropins is continued for 5 to 7 days and then increased by 1 ampule. This procedure is repeated until the effective daily dose (EDD), i.e. the dose which causes a significant and steady estrogen rise, is achieved. In patients with low endogenous estrogens at the initiation of therapy, cervical score examinations may replace estrogen assays for the estimation of EDD. From this day on, the patient is examined daily or on alternate days.

When estrogen levels reach or exceed 250 pg/ml, ultrasonography is performed. If estrogens increase too rapidly or if the day-to-day difference exceeds the geometric rise, the dose is reduced by 1 ampule (75 IU FSH) and treatment is continued at this reduced dose. If the estrogen rise is steady and not excessive, the same dosage is continued until a level of between 350 and 1,200 pg/ml is reached. Since the duration of the active phase is 4 to 6 days, this level should be reached within this time limit. At this stage of therapy, the third sonographic scan is performed. If the total number of measurable follicular structures in both ovaries does not exceed 10 and 1 to 4 follicles have a diameter exceeding 17 mm, the ovulatory dose of hCG (10,000 IU) is administered.

The patient is advised to have sexual intercourse on 3 consecutive days starting on the day of hCG administration. After induction of ovulation, the patient is examined 3 to 5 and 7 to 9 days following the hCG injection. Special care has to be taken not to overlook possible ovarian enlargement, abdominal pains, tenderness or distention, and weight gain exceeding 3 kg. At least one blood sample is drawn and sent for a progesterone assay. The patient is instructed to report back to the clinic if abdominal pains, sudden weight gain, nausea, vomiting, or diarrhea appear. If a sustained high phase of BBT lasts for more than 14 days, an hCG and progesterone assay should be performed.

No consensus has been reached with regard to exogenous hormonal support of the corpus luteum function following induction of ovulation. Some authors advice to support the corpus luteum by 2 or 3 booster injections of 2,500-5,000 IU of hCG on days 5 and 7 after ovulation induction. This is based on two factors: the half-life of exogenous hCG is 6 to 8 hours and the endogenous hCG secreted by the trophoblast becomes detectable from day 7 or 9 following ovulation. The additional hCG injections may be of special importance in patients of Group I and following combined GnRH analog/gonadotropin therapy.

Clinical research and experience showed that, in gonadotropin therapy, multifollicular and multiluteal cycles are the rule rather than an exception (Insler & Potashnik, 1983). However, only a small portion of the multiluteal cycles also results in multiple clinical pregnancies. Brown (1986) remarked that, although multiple preovulatory follicles were seen by ultrasound in 50% of gonadotropin-induced cycles, the recorded multiple pregnancy rate was only 20%. O'Herlihy et al. (1981) showed that multiple preovulatory follicles were found in 71% of clomiphene cycles, but the incidence of multiple pregnancy was only 14%. It is thus probable that in hMG/FSH-induced conception cycles, a number of ova are usually released and possibly fertilized but only one or two of them are destined to produce a viable fetus.

The IVF programs introduced a very important contribution to the management of gonadotropin therapy, particularly when multiple follicles are stimulated. Some of the excessive follicles may be punctured under ultrasound control, thus reducing the E2 levels, leaving a smaller number of follicles to be luteinized by the hCG administration and diminishing the chance of clinical hyperstimulation (Hazout & Belaisch-Allart, 1986).

COMPLICATIONS OF GONADOTROPHIN THERAPY

All complications of gonadotropin treatment are essentially due to ovarian stimulation, follicular development, and luteinization or ovulation. To the best of our knowledge, direct side effects to the drug itself have not been reported. The main complications of gonadotropin treatment are:

1. Ovarian hyperstimulation syndrome
2. High incidence of multiple pregnancy
3. Abortion rate higher than in spontaneous conceptions

Ovarian Hyperstimulation

Introduction and Classification

Ovarian hyperstimulation is the most serious complication of ovulation-induction therapy. The syndrome (OHSS) occurs when ovulation-inducing treatment results in the growth of multiple large follicles followed by the development of follicular and luteal cysts. A comprehensive classification of hyperstimulation into six grades was originally proposed by Rabau et al. (1967) and was later modified into three grades (WHO, 1976) (Table 7–3).

Grade I (mild hyperstimulation) is characterized by variable ovarian enlargement with cysts measuring up to 5 cm in diameter. Laboratory findings include urinary estrogen over 150 μg/24 hrs and pregnanediol excretion exceeding 10 mg/24 hrs. With measurements of steroids in blood this would correspond to E2 values greater than 1,500 pg/ml and progesterone levels over 30 ng/ml in the early luteal phase.

Grade II (moderate hyperstimulation) is characterized by ovarian cysts accompanied by additional symptoms such as abdominal distention, nausea, vomiting, and diarrhea. A sudden weight increase exceeding 3,000 g may be an early sign of moderate hyperstimulation.

Grade III (severe hyperstimulation) is defined by the presence of large ovarian cysts, ascites, and sometimes hydrothorax. Severe hemoconcentration is usually also observed and may, in extreme cases, result in blood hypercoagulation.

Tulandi et al. (1984) found the pregnancy rate in hyperstimulated cycles to be 3 times greater than in nonhyperstimulated cycles. It is generally agreed that mild hyperstimulation (multifollicular development) is associated with an increased pregnancy rate. However, we have shown that in severe hyperstimulation, the abortion rate is significantly higher.

Pathogenesis

Ovarian hyperstimulation is the result of massive follicular luteinization. It therefore occurs only following hCG administration or following an endogenous LH peak induced by the elevated estrogen production of multifollicular growth. In the former case, clinical symptoms usually appear 5 to 10 days following the first dose of hCG. In the latter case, hyperstimulation is extremely rare because the intraovarian regulatory mechanisms and the endogenous negative feedback are usually able to prevent an endogenous LH-surge and therefore massive luteinization does not occur. Ovarian enlargement (with or without cyst formation) and ovulation may occur. Thus, preventing ovulation by withholding hCG is an effective method of avoiding hyperstimulation in overstimulated ovaries.

The fact that ovulation (luteinization) is a precondition necessary for hyperstimulation to occur suggests the involvement of ovarian (corpus luteal) secretions in the pathogenesis of this syndrome. Polishuk & Schenker (1969) found that high-dose hMG treatment caused no complications in male rabbits while all hyperstimulated female rabbits, including a group with extraperitonealized ovaries, displayed ovarian enlargement and ascites. They concluded that ovarian secretion is responsible for increased capillary permeability, causing an extraperitoneal fluid shift. In fact, in severe cases of clinical hyperstimulation, high levels of hormones have been detected, including estradiol, estriol, progesterone, 17-OH-progesterone, pregnanediol, pregnanetriol, testosterone, 17-hydrocorticosteroids, 17-ketosteroids, and aldosterone

TABLE 7-3. Grading of Hyperstimulation

Symptom	Grade I	Grade II	Grade III
Excessice steroid production	+	+	+
Ovarian enlargement	+	+	+
Abdominal discomfort	?	+	+
Ovarian cysts		+	+
Abdominal distension		+	+
Nausea		+	+
Vomiting		+	+
Diarrhea		?	+
Ascites			+
Hydrothorax			+
Severe haemoconcentration			+
Thromboembolic phenomena			?

(Engel et al. 1972; Schenker et al. 1977). The exact factors responsible for enhanced capillary permeability are the subject of debate. Prostaglandins, histamine, and estrogens have been suggested (Schenker and Polishuk, 1976; Engel et al. 1972; Davis, 1960). More recent studies (Navot et al. 1987) seem to indicate that some compounds belonging to the angiotensins system may damage the integrity of capillaries.

Vascular neogenesis is a *conditio sine qua non* of normal follicular growth. In ovarian hyperstimulation syndrome, this process is both enhanced and disturbed, resulting in incompetent capillary function, which leads to re-compartmentialization of body fluids and consequently to a reduction of intravascular volume and the formation of ascites and/or hydrothorax and general edema. Figure 7–7 illustrates the pathogenesis of the ovarian hyperstimulation syndrome.

Regardless of its exact etiology, the increased capillary permeability results in massive ascites and hypovolemia which Engel et al. (1972) term the "cardinal events" in the pathogenesis of the OHSS. Hypovolemia is associated with hemoconcentration, decreased central venous pressure, low blood pressure, and tachycardia. Severe hypovolemia also causes decreased renal perfusion leading to increased reabsorption of sodium and water in the proximal tubule (Polishuk and Schenker, 1969), causing oliguria and low urinary sodium. The exchange of hydrogen and potassium for sodium in the distal tubule is reduced, resulting in an accumulation of H+ and K+, causing hyperkalcemia and a tendency to acidosis (Engel et al. 1972).

The extensiveness of ascites is reflected in the patients' weight gain. Patients with severe OHSS can gain as much as 15–20 kg.

A quite dangerous although extremely rare side effect of OHSS is the occurrence of thromboembolic phenomena. The connection between hMG treatment and clotting abnormalities was first speculated by Mozes et al. (1965). While the cause of thromboembolic phenomena is still not fully established, it is probably related to hemoconcentration (and to elevated estrogen levels). Phillips et al. (1975) reported high levels of factor V, platelets, fibrinogen, profibrinolysin, fibrinolytic inhibitors, and increased thromboplastin generation in patients with OHSS.

Treatment

Since hyperstimulation is a self-limiting disease, its treatment should be symptomatic and conservative even though the severity of its symptoms would seem to demand radical, surgical care. Treatment is generally medical, with laparotomy reserved for cases of an abdominal catastrophe (i.e. ovarian torsion or rupture and internal hemorrhage). The ovarian cysts are so large and brittle that surgical attempts as a palliative procedure usually result in oophorectomy.

Medical treatment of severe hyperstimulation is aimed at: 1) maintaining blood volume while correcting the disturbed fluid and electrolyte balance, 2) preventing thromboembolic phenomena, and 3) relieving secondary complications of hydro-thorax. The patient should be monitored by fluid intake/output records, weight, and frequent measurements of the degree of hemoconcentration as indicated by hemoglobin and hematocrit estimation. In very severe cases, constant measurement of central venous pressure may be indicated. Plasma expanders such as dextran and plasma supplemented with appropriate electrolytes should be administered early.

Diuretic agents are contraindicated since fluid in the third space is unavailable for diuresis and most diuretics influence the distal tubule with minimal effect on the proximal tubule (Engel et al. 1972). Thus, artificially induced diuresis may further

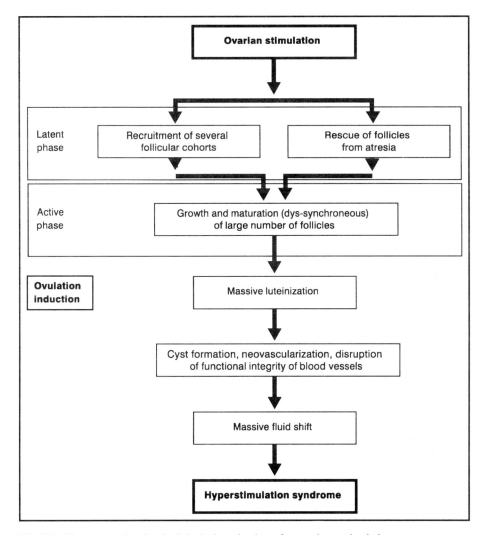

Fig. 7-7. The proposed pathophysiological mechanism of severe hyperstimulation.

diminish the intravascular volume but be unable to cause reduction of the ascites or hydrothorax. Anticoagulant therapy is usually unnecessary if the aforementioned steps are employed promptly. However, due to the danger of disseminated intravascular clotting, blood coagulation should be monitored and, if severe hyper-coagulability is present, heparin treatment may be considered. Since in such cases mini-heparinization is not effective, full heparinization (according to patient's response) should be applied. It should be remembered, however, that in early pregnancy heparin may cause retrotrophoblastic bleeding and lead to abortion.

The third goal of treatment is to relieve pulmonary and/or abdominal symptoms. Pleural effusions should be drained, and Rabau et al. (1967) proposed paracentesis for alleviating breathing difficulty.

Schenker and Weinstein (1978) argue against paracentesis because of the danger of puncturing cysts and causing intraperitoneal hemorrhage. In our hands, paracentesis did not cause intraperitoneal hemorrhage. Needless to say, puncturing the abdominal cavity and/or ovarian cysts should be performed under sonographic control.

Incidence of Hyperstimulation

Analysis of several large series encompassing 11,342 cycles of treatment showed that the incidence of moderate and severe hyperstimulation was 3.4%, and 0.84% respectively (Table 7–4). It should be noted that all the above reports included cases treated without sonographic monitoring. The influence of patients' selection, treatment schedules, and monitoring methods on the relative risks of hyperstimulation have been discussed in previous sections (see: Selection of patients, Treatment schemes, and Monitoring of therapy). It is true that only some of the patients who received hCG, despite inappropriate rise or excessive levels of estrogen, developed ovarian hyperstimulation. Only future statistical analysis will demonstrate whether or not the additional use of sonography will enable a further reduction in the rate of hyperstimulation or multiple births.

TABLE 7–4. Incidence of ovarian Hyperstimulation in Gonadotropin-induced Cycles

Authors	Year	No. of Cycles	Percent of Cycles with Hyperstimulation	
			Mild	Severe
Thompson & Hansen	1970	2 798	?	1.3
Spadoni et al.	1974	225	4.4	1.8
Ellis & Williamson	1975	322	5.0	0.6
Caspi et al.	1976	343	6.0	1.2
Australian Department of Health	1981	4 008	3.7	0.9
Lunenfeld et al.	1982	3 646	3.1	0.25
Total		11 343	3.4	0.84

Multiple Pregnancy

Multiple pregnancy is rather frequent following gonadotropin therapy. Brown (1986) reviewed 1,712 pregnancies resulting from ovulation-induction by human pituitary or menopausal gonadotropins and found that the average multiple pregnancy rate was 24.4%, fluctuating between 21 and 33%. As expected, small series showed lower incidence of multiple gestations than large series. The causes of multiple conceptions following induced cycles are very similar to the causes of ovarian hyperstimulation, i.e. the pharmacological stimulation of multifollicular development. Thus, the risk factors and the possibilities to avoid (or at least reduce the incidence) of both complications are similar (see section on Ovarian hyperstimulation). Insler & Potashnik (1983) reported that, in 26% of gonadotropin-induced cycles, three or more functional corpora lutea were produced, and that mean plateau progesterone levels were higher in the conceptional than in the non-conceptional cycles. Further analysis of the above mentioned data indicated that, in hMG treatment cycles, conception occurs in most cases in the presence of more than one corpus luteum and, in 25% of the cases, in the presence of three or more functioning corpora lutea. Since only around 25% of gonadotropin-induced pregnancies result in twins and only 5% produce three or more fetuses, and since the mean plateau progesterone levels are similar in single and multiple hMG-induced pregnancies, it could be speculated that in the majority of hMG/FSH conceptions a number of ova are released and fertilized but only one of them is destined to produce a living fetus. The others perish before reaching the uterine cavity or are absorbed or extruded prior to implantation.

If, however, a quadruplet, quintuplet etc., pregnancy reaches the gestational age of 7 to 8 weeks, its further development may represent a severe danger to the fetuses because of a very high probability of extreme prematurity, a considerable medical complication to the mother, and a pronounced psychological, social, and financial burden to the family. The technique of fetal reduction under sonographic control has been developed. Breckwoldt et al. (1988) reported a case of gonadotropin-induced pregnancy with 9 gestational sacks present in the uterus. Six of the fetuses were eliminated under sonographic guidance. This technique, although medically simple and logical, is still controversial for ethical, legal, and religious reasons.

Abortions

The abortion rate in conceptions following gonadotrophin therapy is around 21%. Brown (1986) compiled and reviewed a series of 1,712 pregnancies and found that the combined abortion and perinatal deaths rates fluctuated from 10 % to 28 % in different reports.

There was no significant difference in the abortion rate between diagnostic groups. The rate was 26% in patients of Group I and 32.6% in women of Group II, respectively (Blankstein et al. 1986). However, the abortion rate in the first conception cycle (28.8%) was significantly higher than in the second or third gestation (12.8%). The main reasons for increased abortion rates in conceptions resulting from induction of ovulation are probably as follows:

a) luck of structural, genetic, and functional integrity of the zygote;
b) structural and functional inadequacy of the endometrium in ensuring proper and timely nidation of the embryo;
c) functional incompetence of the corpus luteum preventing it from a proper reaction to the pregnancy signal, i.e. different peptides and hCG produced by the fertilized egg;
d) multiple pregnancy;
e) emotional factors;
f) exessive LH levels in the late follicular phase.

CONCEPTION RATES

Conception rates following gonadotropin therapy are dependent on the following factors (in order of importance):

   * selection of patients
  ** type of monitoring
*** treatment scheme

In women with hypothalamic-pituitary failure (Group I), substitution therapy with gonadotropins is very efficient in inducing ovulation and pregnancy. Gonadotropin treatment applied as a stimulation therapy in patients having some albeit deranged hypothalamic-pituitary-gonadal function (Group II), is by far more complicated and less efficient (see Section: Treatment schemes).

While in patients of Group I pregnancy rates of up to 82% were achieved, in Group II conception rates varied between 20% and 35% (Lunenfeld & Insler, 1978; Lunenfeld et al. 1985; Australian Department of Health, 1981; Bettendorf et al. 1981a). The same discrepancy was also seen when cumulative pregnancy rates were calculated using the life-table analysis method. In Group I, after 6 cycles of therapy, the cumulative pregnancy rate exceeded 90%. In contrast, patients of Group II required 12 cycles of therapy in order to reach a cumulative conception rate of less than 60%.

The age of the patients also markedly influences the outcome of treatment. Women over 35 years of age had a significantly reduced conception rate, regardless of the type of diagnosis and treatment (Insler et al. 1981a). The duration of amenorrhea, on the other hand, had no bearing on the results of gonadotropin therapy. The treatment was as efficient in women who were amenorrheic for one year only as in those who suffered from amenorrhea for 10 years or more.

Table 7–5 shows the results of gonadotropin therapy as reported by 16 different groups working independently on 4 continents. This list does not purport to include all data on gonadotropin therapy published so far. It nevertheless shows the overall dimension of this therapy and its importance in the therapeutic armamentarium of fertility clinics throughout the world. The list includes more than 22,000 courses of treatment given to 8,036 women and almost 3,000 conceptions. Since the majority of entries deals with rather large groups of patients, this summary represents the results of gonadotropin treatment in unselected material typical of busy fertility clinics.

The pregnancy rates (per patient) varied between 23.1% and 82.5%, with an average of 34.7%. Pregnancy rates per cycle ranged from 7.1% to 22.5%. The intensity of treatment (the mean number of courses of treatment per patient) fluctuated from 2.0 to 4.2. Knowing the pregnancy rate per cycle specific to each clinic, one can easily calculate the overall prognosis and the cost of this treatment.

OUTCOME OF PREGNANCIES

The course of gestation following the induction of ovulation with hMG appears to be normal. Analysis of the mode of delivery showed a high incidence of interventions, breech extraction, vacuum extraction, forceps delivery, and cesarean sections. The high incidence of obstetrical intervention may be explained by multiple pregnancy rate, primiparity ratios, and psychological factors involved in delivering a "premium child" in patients of long-standing infertility. Our study (Lunenfeld et al. 1987) showed that the sex ratio (M/F) of the single births was 1.06 (54% boys) and of the twins 0.72 (42% boys). The number of triplets was too small to analyze. In 1976, Caspi reported 32 males and 50 females in the single births (39%) with a twin M/F ratio of 0.78 (Caspi et al. 1976). In the series reported by Bettendorf et al. (1981a), the incidence of male children in single pregnancies was 51.8%. However, in the above author's series, the incidence of male children in twins and triplets was 53.8% and 66.7%, respectively. The normal secondary sex ratio at 28 weeks is considered to be 106 boys to 100 girls (Tricomi et al. 1960; Serr and Ismajovich, 1963).

TABLE 7-5. Conception rates following gonadotrophin therapy

Authors (Year)	Patients	Cycles	Number	Pregnancies % Cycles	% Pat.
Butler (1970)	134	438	31	7.1	23.1
Gemzell (1970)	228	463	101	21.8	44.3
Thompson & Hansen (1970)	1190	2798	334	11.9	28.1
Caspi et al. (1974)	101	343	62	18.1	61.4
Spadoni et al. (1974)	62	225	26	11.5	41.9
Ellis & Williamson (1975)	77	332	43	13.3	55.8
Tsapoulis et al. (1978)	320	?	163		50.9
Healy et al. (1980)	40	159	33	20.7	82.5
Australian Department of Health (1981)	1056	4008	552	13.8	52.3
Bettendorf et al. (1981a)	756	1585	224	14.1	29.6
Goldfarb et al. (1982)	442	1098	118	10.7	26.7
Kurachi (1983)	2166	6096	523	8.6	24.2
Lunenfeld et al. (1985)	1107	3646	424	11.6	38.3
Tuang (1985)	95	320	72	22.5	75.8
Potashnik et al. (1986)	262	580	85	14.6	32.4
Total	8036	> 22 000	2791		34.7

The sex ratio (M/F) for twins was found by Nichols (1952) to be 1.043, for triplets 1.007 and for quadruplets 0.940. The high incidence of girls in our twin series and the high incidence of male children in twins and triplets in the series of Bettendorf et al. (1981a) are probably due to the rather small numbers involved. By combining all the 3 series, one approaches the expected sex ratios clearly indicating the importance of sufficiently large numbers in order to estimate similarities or divergence in sex ratio.

Congenital Malformations

Table 7-6 shows the rate of congenital malformations found in a combined series of 941 babies born after induction of ovulation with hMG/hCG. The incidence was 22.3/1,000 and 19.1/1,000 for minor and major malformation respectively. The

TABLE 7-6. Congenital Malformations

Authors (Year)	No.	Major	Minor
Caspi et al. (1976)	157	4	11
Harlap (1976)	66	1	5
Hack and Lunenfeld (1978)	209	4	4
Kurachi et al. (1983)	509	9	1
Total	941	18 (1.91)	21 (2.23)
Normal Population		1.27 (0.31–2.25)	7.24

incidence of congenital malformations in normal populations has been reported to be 12.7/1,000 after 28 weeks gestation, with a range of 3.1 to 22.5 (Stevenson et al. 1966; McKeown, 1960). There is a further rise to 23.1/1,000 by the age of 5 years. Hendricks (1966) reported a rate of 3% in the neonatal period, with twice as many malformations in twin births, mostly monozygotic twins. The clinical evidence does not indicate that babies born after hMG/hCG ovulation induction are at any greater risk of malformation than the general population.

LONG-TERM SAFETY

Nulliparity has been a consistently reported risk factor for carcinoma of the breast and endometrium (Ron et al. 1985; Kelsey, 1979; Kelsey et al. 1982; Brinton et al. 1983; LaVecchia et al. 1984). With regard to cancer incidence among the 1,438 functionally infertile patients in our series (Lunenfeld et al. 1987), the rate of hormone-associated tumors was 1.5 times the expected rate. For carcinoma of the breast, it was 1.4, and for endometrial cancers 8.0 times as high. In an attempt to assess whether risk factors could be linked to different etiologies within this heterogeneous group, these infertile patients were analyzed according to 3 types of infertility:

1) Amenorrheic patients with low endogenous estrogens and gonadotropins (141 women)
2) Infertile women displaying both estrogens and postovulatory progesterone whose infertility was due to mechanical factors, male factor, or unexplained infertility (712 patients)
3) Amenorrheic or anovulatory patients displaying endogenous estrogens but lacking or having less than normal postovulatory progesterone (992 patients)

In the amenorrheic group of 141 patients with low endogenous estrogens and gonadotropins, the observed hormone-associated cancer rate was lower than the expected rate for all sites. Not a single case of breast, endometrial, or other hormone-associated cancers was detected (although 1.68 were expected) in patients of this group, regardless of whether hMG/hCG therapy was followed by pregnancy or not.

In the 712 women with infertility due to mechanical or male factors and displaying both estrogen and postovulatory progesterone, no increased risk for hormone-associated cancers was observed.

In the 992 amenorrheic or anovulatory women who had fluctuating estrogen levels but lacked sufficient postovulatory progesterone, the observed rate of uterine and breast cancer was 10.3 and 1.8 times the expected rate (Table 7-7).

TABLE 7-7. Observed (Obs.) and Expected (Exp.) Breast and Uterine Cancers in Infertile Patients

	No.	Breast			Uterus		
		Obs.	Exp.	Obs./Exp.	Obs.	Exp.	Obs./Exp.
Estrogen (–) Progesterone (–)	141	0	1.02	–	0	0.09	–
Estrogen + Progesterone +	712	3	4.57	0.7	0	0.37	–
Estrogen + Progesterone (–)	992	8	4.43	1.8	3	0.29	10.3

Of the above group, 385 women were treated with hMG/hCG. 198 conceived and in 187 cases no record of conception exists. In the former group, not a single case of breast or uterine cancer was observed. On the other hand, in the 187 women who failed to conceive, the observed breast and uterine cancer rate was 2.83 and 28.57 times higher than the expected rates, respectively (Table 7-8).

TABLE 7-8. Observed (Obs.) and Expected (Exp.) Breast and Uterine Cancers following Induction of Ovulation with hMG/hCG

	No.	Breast			Uterus		
		Obs.	Exp.	Obs./Exp.	Obs.	Exp.	Obs./Exp.
No Pregnancy	187	3	1.06	2.83	2	0.07	28.57
Conceptions	198	0	1.07	–	0	0.07	–

The above data indicate that hMG/hCG therapy does not increase the risk of cancer. Because the number of women receiving each specific treatment is small and the majority of patients has not yet reached the age of the maximal cancer risk, the statistical power to detect minor effects of treatment was low. However, a large cancer risk would certainly have been detected. It seems from the results presented that, among infertile patients, only anovulatory women with unopposed estrogens are at increased risk for uterine and breast cancer. Induction of ovulation in these patients with hMG/hCG followed by conception seems to reduce the risk.

Induction of ovulation with human gonadotropins is a well-established therapeutic method. Its efficacy is unequivocal in women with hypothalamic-pituitary failure (Group I). In patients with hypothalamic-pituitary dysfunction (Group II), gonadotropin treatment, however less efficient than in Group I, represents an additional therapeutic possibility over and above that offered by other ovulation-inducing agents. New insights provided by the introduction of sonography and IVF and the constant search for better treatment schemes, such as combined GnRH analogs/gonadotropin therapy, constitute a firm basis for the prediction that, in the near future, gonadotropin therapy will become as efficient in Group II as it is now in Group I.

8. THE CERVICAL FACTOR

Spermatozoa must traverse a long and complicated path through the female genital tract in order to reach and subsequently penetrate a fertilizable egg. In order to ensure proper reproduction rates, Nature has developed a multifactorial, complex system of protecting sperm cells during their passage from the vagina to the Fallopian tube.

One of the main components of this system is the uterine cervix. The main functions of the uterine cervix and its secretion in the conception process are:

1. Protection of sperm from the hostile environment of the vagina
2. Supplementation of the energy requirements of spermatozoa
3. Facilitation of sperm passage from the vagina into the uterus during the periovulatory period and interference with sperm transport at all other times
4. Selective filtration of morphologically abnormal spermatozoa and impedance of their progress to the upper parts of the female genital tract
5. Preservation of viable spermatozoa within the cervical crypts and their successive release into the uterus. This function ensures the availability of viable sperm over a prolonged period of time following ejaculation and prevents overcrowding of spermatozoa at the impregnation site.

The uterine cervix is well-equipped for exercising its complicated and important function.

ANATOMY AND PHYSIOLOGY

In the human, the cervix is a cylindrical structure several centimeters long. It is composed mainly of muscular and fibrous tissue. Approximately at its center, the cervix is bored through by a longitudinal duct called the endocervical canal. The proximal end of the endocervical canal (internal cervical os) opens into the uterine cavity, and the distal end (external cervical os) is situated in the upper part of the vagina. The external cervical os usually points toward the posterior vaginal fornix. Following ejaculation, the external os of the cervix is immersed in the seminal fluid that is pooled in the posterior vaginal fornix.

The endocervical canal is lined by a mucus membrane forming an intricate system of invaginations, folds, and recesses called the cervical crypts (Fig. 8-1). It is the inner space of the cervical crypt that provides for the storage of spermatozoa and it is the secretory unit of the cervical epithelium that produces the secretion vital for sperm support and transport.

The cervical crypts, i.e. pockets and folds of the columnar epithelium, may run in various directions – longitudinal, oblique or transverse to the axis of the uterine cervix. They may bifurcate or side branch, but do not, as a rule, cross each other. The number, size, and location of the cervical crypts vary with age and are influenced by the hormonal milieu prevailing at various phases of the menstrual cycle. According to Odeblad (1966), the endocervical canal contains some 100 mucus-secreting units (crypts). Our own research (Bernstein et al. 1977) indicates that the number of cervical crypts is much larger, comprising several thousand units with a total circumference of several meters.

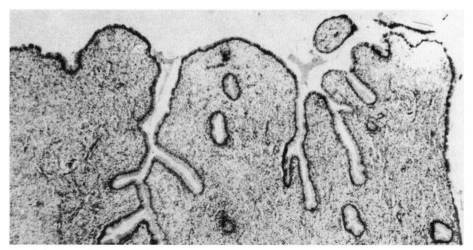

Fig. 8-1. Microphotograph of a section through the endocervical epithelium. Note that the cervical crypts extend in different directions running longitudinally, obliquely or transversly to the lumen.

The endocervical mucosa consists of several types of nonciliated secretory cells and of ciliated cells (Fig. 8-2). The nonciliated secretory cells contain many cytoplasmic granules which may push the nucleus out of its central position toward the basal membrane. During the secretory phase, the cell membrane ruptures and the secretory granules (components of the cervical mucus) are released into the lumen of the endocervical canal (Hafez, 1973a). According to Chilton's elegant studies in the rabbit (Chilton et al. 1980a; 1980b), more than one population of mucus-producing cells exist in the endocervix. The number and function of these cells depend on the hormonal milieu. The mucus-producing cell populations are significantly diminished in ovariectomized animals but may be restored by the application of exogenous

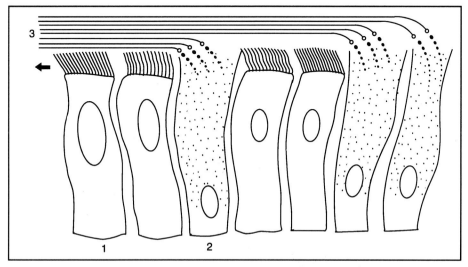

Fig. 8-2. Schematic picture of different cell types of the cervical mucosa: 1 = ciliated cell, 2 = secretory cell, 3 = cervical mucus. The direction of cilia beat is indicated by an arrow.

estrogens. Histochemical studies (Gaton et al. 1982) showed that the same crypt may produce different types of mucus and that, even within the same cell, more than one type of glycoproteins may be synthesized.

Ciliated cells are interspersed, singly or in groups, between the secretory cells. The proportion of ciliated cells to secretory cells differs in various parts of the cervix. Within the endocervix, the relation is one ciliated cell per 20 secretory elements (Jordan and Allen, 1977). According to Gaton et al. (1982), the secretory cells represent up to 78% of the total cell population in the endocervix. Large crypts contain more secretory cells than small crypts and the number of functioning secretory cells is dependent on the amount of estrogens and gestagens and their ratio. The luminal surface of the ciliated cells is covered with a dense layer of kinocilia. The kinocilia beat toward the vagina and probably play a role in the orientation of macromolecules and in the direction of flow of the mucus produced by the secretory elements (see Fig. 8.2). Ciliated cells may undergo deciliation. The stimulus triggering this process is still unknown. After menopause, a certain degree of deciliation usually takes place (Hafez, 1973b).

The mucus membrane of the human cervix does not reflect ovarian cyclicity as accurately as does the endometrium (Davies and Woolf, 1961; Friedrich, 1973; Fand, 1973). However, both the length and diameter of the endocervical canal (Insler et al. 1970; Mann et al. 1961), as well as the number and size of the cervical crypts, exhibit definite changes throughout the menstrual cycle (Bernstein et al. 1977). It seems that estrogen stimulation increases the number of crypts in the lower cervix and the mean size of crypts in the upper cervix, thus significantly enlarging the spermatozoal storage space. There is no doubt that the secretory activity of the cervical epithelium is governed by hormonal changes. The daily production of mucus varies between 20 mg at the beginning and at the end of the cycle, and 600 mg at midcycle (Matsumoto, 1962; Macdonald, 1969; Elstein, 1970). The actual amount of mucus and its compositions is a function of the number of crypts and the level and ratio of sex steroids.

COMPOSITION OF THE CERVICAL MUCUS

Cervical mucus is a mixture of uterine, tubal, and possibly follicular fluids, blood transudate, and secretion of the cervical epithelium. Chemical constituents and, consequently, physical properties of the mucus undergo dramatic changes during the menstrual cycle in response to different levels and ratios of estrogenic and progestational hormones. The cervical mucus is a hydrogel composed of a matrix or high-viscosity component and of cervical plasma or a low-viscosity component (Gibbons and Mattner, 1971; Doehr and Moghissi, 1973). Both components are very rich in water, which makes up some 85–99% of the mucus (Odeblad, 1973; Macdonald, 1969). Water acts as the hydrating medium for the high-viscosity insoluble protein matrix and as a vehicle for soluble molecules of the cervical plasma. Estrogen increases and progesterone diminishes the water content of the cervical mucus.

Soluble Constituents of the Cervical Mucus

The soluble constituents of the cervical mucus are numerous and of different types (Gibbons & Mattner, 1971; Elstein & Daunter, 1973; Weed & Carrera, 1970;

Iacobelli et al. 1971). Inorganic salts (mainly NaCl, potassium, copper, zinc, magnesium, calcium, phosphate, sulfate, and bicarbonate), low molecular compounds such as glucose, maltose, and mannose, proteins, peptides, and lipids were found in the cervical mucus. The main task of all these components is to provide a proper medium for the preservation and migration of the sperm. Soluble proteins making up some 30% of the nondialysable material of the cervical mucus gel may either constitute a local cervical secretion or may originate from higher parts of the genital tract, or may even be produced by cells migrating into the cervical mucus.

Soluble cervical mucus proteins have been extensively studied by Schumacher, Moghissi and Elstein and their coworkers (Moghissi & Neuhaus, 1966; Schumacher, 1971, 1973a, 1973b; Schill & Schumacher, 1973; Elstein, 1970). It is logical to assume that at least part of the proteins found in the cervical mucus reach it by transudation from blood. However, the cervical epithelium is apparently able to synthesize and secrete protein material. Labeled amino acids have been incorporated into IgA and IgG in human cervical tissue cultures. IgG- and IgM-producing plasma cells have been identified in the cervical tissue. The fact that the cervical mucus may contain immunoglobulins, i.e. specific antibodies, either transudated from the plasma or locally produced (Hulka & Omran, 1969), is of great interest and clinical significance. This finding indicates that, under certain conditions, locally produced antibodies could impede fertility by interfering with sperm migration or vitality (Behrman, 1968; Shulman, 1972). All the soluble proteins of the cervical mucus, including enzymes and immunoglobulins, are probably subject to cycle variations in response to hormonal stimuli. This fact could be of practical value in the detection of approaching ovulation and certainly is of great physiological significance in the conception process.

It seems that the concentration of soluble proteins in the cervical mucus is at its lowest at midcycle (Krumme et al. 1977). The importance of this finding in the physiology of conception and its possible application to contraception are obvious.

Insoluble Protein Matrix of the Cervical Mucus

The chemical structure and properties of the insoluble cervical mucus macromolecular proteins were studied in depth by Pigman and Moschera (1973), Gibbons and Sellwood (1973), Syner and Moghissi (1971), Masson (1973), and Bhushana Rao and Masson (1977). Valuable information about the properties of cervical mucus gel was added by the scanning electron microscopy studies of Hafez et al. (1975), Chretien (1977), and Elstein and Daunter (1977).

The core of the cervical mucus determining its gel-like appearance and, to a great extent, its physical and rheological properties is a macromolecule called mucin. It is composed of protein containing more than 40% carbohydrates distributed along the peptide core in the form of numerous side chains. Mucin macromolecules form bundles with a thickness of about $0.5-1.5$ μm. The size of these bundles corresponds to the diameter of secretory granules found in the nonciliated cells of the cervical epithelium. The carbohydrate side chains consist of a number of different sugars like fucose, galactose, sialic acid, etc. In individuals possessing the secretor gene, the oligosaccharides may possess the specific structure of AB0 blood group activity. Bhushana Rao and Masson (1977) suggested that the mucin filaments are actually composed of repeated subunits with a molecular weight of about 30,000 daltons, possibly linked by hydrophobic bonds. Each subunit consists of two parts which differ in composition and size. The major part consists of 19 amino acid residues and contains all the carbohydrates of the subunit. The minor segment is devoid of carbohydrate side chains. The mucin filaments form a network in which individual filaments are held together by disulfide bridges.

The viscosity and coherence of the mucins is due to the rigidity of the mucin macromolecule and to the multiple interconnections between the threadlike individual molecules. Cyclic changes of the rheological properties of the cervical mucus such as viscosity, threadability, tack, etc., may be explained by changes in the mucin/soluble proteins ratio, the density of intermolecular linkages, and modification of the carbohydrate composition of the chains.

The production of mucin is stimulated by estrogen, but the final rheological properties of the mucus depend on the estrogen/progestin ratio which, on the one hand, determines the amount of mucus and, on the other hand, may render it more or less viscous and thick, depending on the amount of water hydrating the macromolecular core and on the concentration of soluble protein. Both latter functions are under hormonal control, which is exerted on the mucus-producing cells in the crypts, the cervical stroma, and also on the capillaries bordering the cervical crypts.

It should be noted that the bulk of cervical mucus found in the lumen of the endocervical canal differs from the mucus produced by the epithelial cells within the crypts (Gaton et al. 1982). This suggests that the cervical stromal tissue plays an important role in mucus production and in the determination of its content. In a series of elegant in vivo and in vitro experiments in the rabbit, Nicosia (1981) showed that there is a close relationship between mucus production and the blood flow within the capillaries as well as the permeability of the microvessels walls in the endocervical stroma. He also indicated that blood serum contains a powerful, nonhormonal inducer of mucus granules-release by the endocervical secretory cells. Moreover, water, electrolytes, soluble proteins, and other substances transudated from blood vessels define the final composition of cervical mucus and, consequently, its physical and rheological properties as well as its biological function, i.e. sperm penetrability.

TYPES OF CERVICAL MUCUS

The physical, rheological, and biological properties of the intraluminar cervical mucus and their changes during the menstrual cycle were studied by different methods. The Swedish group led by Odeblad employed the magnetic resonance method (Odeblad, 1973; Hoeglund & Odeblad, 1977). Lee et al. (1977) used light-scattering spectroscopy. Others applied scanning electron microscopy (Hafez et al. 1975; Chretien, 1977; Elstein & Daunter, 1977). Several other groups studied the properties of the cervical mucus using biological and clinical means (Insler et al. 1972; Reichman et al. 1973a, 1973b; Kerin et al. 1976). These different approaches produced a rather complete and concise understanding of the various functions and properties of cervical mucus.

It has been noted that there exist two types of mucus: The periovulatory mucus (E mucus) reflecting high levels of estrogens unopposed by gestagens, and the scanty mucus (G mucus) produced either in response to very low estrogen levels or when both estrogens and gestagens are present.

Type E Mucus: is thin and watery and consists of 95–98% water, 1% proteins, and 0.5–1.5% glycoproteins. The macromolecular glycoprotein micelles are lying 0.5–5 μm apart from one another with only a few cross-links between them. Owing to the rapid flow, the micelles line up more or less parallel to the axis of the cervical canal. The lines of strain lead from the mucus-producing cells in the cervical crypts toward the external os. This type of mucus prevails around the time of ovulation. At that time, the cervical mucus forms parallel channels with a diameter of approximately 3 μm filled with thin, watery cervical plasma. Sperm cells entering these channels may not only swim freely in the lumen but are also oriented in the proper direction towards the uterine cavity. The sperm are probably propelled upward by minute contractions of the longitudinal micelles forming the walls of the channels.

Moreover, the intermicellar cross-linkage may serve as a ladder facilitating the ascent of spermatozoa into the uterine cavity. Lee et al. (1977) studied human midcycle mucus by light-scattering spectroscopy and concluded that it is composed of an ensemble of loosely entangled, randomly coiled macromolecules rather than of cross-linked, more or less parallel fibrils.

Type G Mucus: is thick and sticky. It contains 85–92% water, 2–4% protein, and 2–10% mucin. Due to extensive cross-linking, the mucin is arranged in a dense network with a mesh size of 0.1–0.5 μm. Since the width of the head of a spermatozoon is 2.5 μm, mucus of type G is virtually impenetrable to sperm. Mucus of this type prevails during the luteal phase of the cycle, following the administration of potent gestagens, and during early pregnancy.

This basic information derived from the extensive studies of Odeblad (1973), Gibbons & Mattner (1971), Davajan et al. (1971), Insler et al. (1972), Hafez et al. (1975), Poon & McCoshen (1985) makes the understanding and interpretation of clinical observations much easier. To complete the picture, it might be useful at this point to briefly recapitulate the basic types of the cervical secretion observed in daily clinical work.

When under strong estrogenic stimulation, i.e. during the periovulatory period or when potent exogenous doses of estrogen are administered, the uterine cervix produces abundant, watery, thin mucus almost free of cell elements, with high threadability and pronounced ferning capacity. The sperm penetrability is highest at this period.

When under the influence of both estrogen and progesterone, i.e. during the luteal phase, under the influence of the combined contraceptive pill, or in pregnancy, the cervical epithelium produces scant, thick mucus of high viscosity and low threadability. At this point, it is almost devoid of ferning capacity and contains many cells. Such mucus is practically impenetrable to sperm. The sperm penetrability of human cervical mucus becomes significant on approximately the 8th day of a normal ovulatory cycle and increases, gradually reaching a peak one day prior to ovulation. Sperm penetration is usually markedly decreased one or two days after ovulation.

MECHANISM OF SPERM MIGRATION
THROUGH THE CERVICAL MUCUS

This subject has been studied in detail by Kremer (1968), Davajan & Kunitake (1969), Sobrero (1974), Kerin et al. (1976), and Insler et al. (1981). The penetration of sperm from the vaginal pool into the uterus is a function of at least 3 different factors:

a) the ability of the cervical secretory units to produce mucus in adequate amount and with the proper physical and rheological properties
b) the nature of the ejaculate, particularly in regard to the number and motility of spermatozoa
c) the number, size, and functional capacity of the cervical crypts.

Normal human ejaculate contains some 100–500 million spermatozoa, which are deposited in the vaginal fornix and on the cervix. The first portion of the ejaculate, containing sperm of the highest concentration and quality, may enter the cervical mucus very promptly. Sobrero & MacLeod (1962) found motile sperm in the endocervical canal 1.5 minutes after ejaculation. The portion of the sperm remaining in the vagina undergoes immediate coagulation. This process probably protects sperm cells from being adversely affected by the low pH of the vaginal surroundings. Additional protection is furnished by the alkaline cervical mucus coating the upper part of the vagina.

Following liquefaction of the coagulate by seminal proteolytic enzymes, the main bulk of the sperm enter the uterine cervix and begin their migration toward the upper part of the female genital tract. Since they possess only a meagre reserve of endogenous glycogen, spermatozoa must depend on extracellular energy sources. While in the seminal plasma, sperm derive the energy required for vital processes and motility from fructose by means of anaerobic fructolysis. After entering the mucus, aerobic metabolism may ensue (Mann, 1973). Cervical secretion is known to contain glycogen, glucose, mannose, and other sugars. Amylase capable of reducing glycogen to glucose has also been found in the cervical secretion. As to the oxygen required for aerobic glycolysis, probably enough of this gas may diffuse from the blood vessels supplying the cervical mucosa.

As mentioned above, the bulk of spermatozoa enters the uterine cavity, passing through the column of the intraluminal mucus. The cervical crypts serve as an important additional mechanism of sperm preservation and transport. Although there is no doubt that endocervical crypts play an important role as a sperm reservoir, the number of spermatozoa stored in the endocervix is rather small (100,000–200,000) (Settlage et al. 1973; Insler et al. 1981).

Crypts situated along the whole length of the cervical canal are colonized by spermatozoa within 2 hours following insemination (Fig. 8–3). Sperm cells are stored mainly in large crypts equipped with a number of side branches. Medium-sized crypts and sometimes even small ones may, however, serve as additional storage facilities. The sperm storage capacity of the endocervix is regulated by sex steroids. Estrogens enlarge the storage space by increasing the number and size of cervical crypts, particularly in the upper cervix. They also affect the mucus-secreting units, the cervical stroma, and the cervical vasculature, resulting in the production of mucus particularly favorable to sperm storage and preservation. Gestagens were shown to have an opposite effect (Insler et al. 1981).

It has been demonstrated (Mattner, 1968) that only motile sperm reach the cervical crypts. Dead sperm are mostly found in the center of the cervical mucus. It should be stressed that, at least in primates, the number of leukocytes found in the central part of the mucus far exceeds that found within the crypts (Jaszczak, 1973). It may be

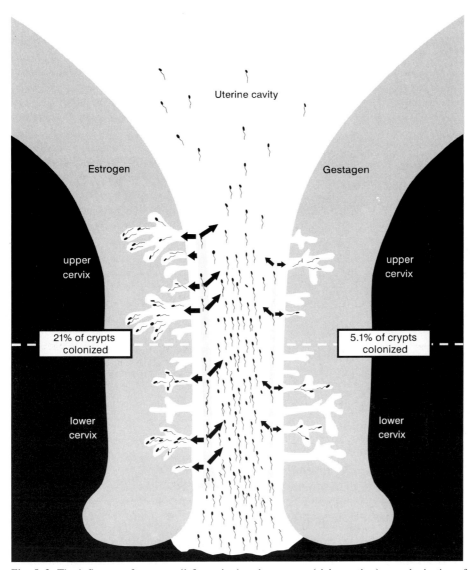

Fig. 8-3. The influence of estrogen (left portion) and gestagens (right portion) on colonization of cervical crypts by spermatozoa.
(From: V. Insler, M. Glezerman, D. Bernstein, L. Zejdel & N. Misgav: Cervical crypts and their role in storing spermatozoa. In: V. Insler, G. Bettendorf & KH. Geissler (Eds.) Advances in diagnosis and treatment of infertility, Elsevier – North Holland, New York, 1981.)

speculated that live sperm resting in the crypts and awaiting their turn to be released into the uterus are protected from phagocytosis, while dead spermatozoa in the central part of the mucus column (being in physical proximity to leukocytes) may be efficiently eliminated. It seems also that abnormal sperm do not migrate through the cervical mucus as efficiently as normal spermatozoa (Perry et al. 1977). In rabbits and in primates, at comparable times following artificial insemination, a higher number of sperm have been recovered from the cervix than from the uterotubal junction (Hafez, 1973b). Moreover, the cervical mucus is undoubtedly one of the best media for the preservation of the life and motility of spermatozoa. Motile sperm have been recovered from the human cervical canal up to 205 hours after coitus (Sobrero, 1974). This mechanism prevents overcrowding of sperm at the impregnation site, makes conception possible even when coitus does not exactly coincide with the discharge of the egg, and prevents abnormal spermatozoa from reaching the ovum.

The above findings strongly seem to suggest that the uterine cervix and its secretion act as both sperm reservoir and sperm selector. The sperm-transporting activity of the cervix is controlled by ovarian steroids. Penetration, density, and speed are greatest in preovulatory mucus (Kremer, 1968; Carlborg et al. 1969). Kerin et al. (1976) narrowed the period of best penetrability to only two days – one day before and the day of LH peak. At all other times, cervical mucus presents a barrier virtually impenetrable to sperm. The physiological explanation for the latter finding is quite obvious. Large numbers of sperm present in the oviduct together with the fertilized egg might unfavorably affect the external milieu of the ovum or the zygote.

CLINICAL APPROACH TO THE EVALUATION
OF THE CERVICAL FACTOR OF INFERTILITY

Pathological conditions rendering any of the complicated functions of the cervix inadequate, may result in disturbed sperm penetration and infertility. According to Moghissi (1973), primary or secondary abnormalities of the cervix or cervical secretion may be responsible for impeded fertility in approximately 15% of all infertile couples. Since methods for the treatment of other factors of infertility became more efficient, the relative importance of the cervical factor has increased.

Whenever clinical evaluation of the cervical factor is attempted, the first problem to be solved is to distinguish between:

1. disturbed ovarian control mechanism
2. disturbed sperm deposition
3. disturbed sperm migration (sperm defect)
4. disturbed sperm transport (mucus defect)

Although all of the above-mentioned disturbances may eventually result in infertility due to reduced sperm penetration, only the last represents *sensu stricto* a disease of the uterine cervix.

At present, several methods are available for screening infertile couples for the presence of disturbed mucus/sperm interaction. The most widely used is the traditional postcoital test (PCT). This test is based on the number of motile spermatozoa per high-power microscopic field in a mucus sample collected some time after coitus. In order to make this evaluation valid, the following four criteria must be met:

a) the mucus has to be of good quality in adequate amount, and the test must be performed immediately after collection of the sample (before the mucus dries)
b) the mucus must be free of contamination with vaginal secretions as far as possible
c) consistent classification of the results must be used

d) details concerning the amount and quality of the cervical mucus, the time interval between coitus and sampling, and the results of the test must be consistently and clearly recorded.

Many different methods have been advocated for the classification of the results of PCT. According to Marcus & Marcus (1965), the test is graded as negative when no sperm cells, motile or dead, are found in the entire mucus specimen; poor when various numbers of sperm are seen but none are motile; fair when up to 6 motile sperm cells are observed; good when 7 to 20 sperm cells are observed; and excellent when more than 20 motile spermatozoa per field are observed. Five to ten high-power fields are counted and the mean number is then calculated.

In 1976, a WHO consulting team suggested a grading system which seems to be simple and useful. The test is considered to be normal when more then seven spermatozoa with good progressive movement are observed per high-power field; inconclusive, when one to seven sperm cells with good motility are present in each field; and abnormal, when either sperm cells are immobilized or not present in the mucus sample.

To be of clinical significance, the PCT has to be repeated several times. We perform the first check some 12 to 16 hours after coitus and, if the result is normal on two occasions, there is no need to repeat the test. If the result is inconclusive or abnormal, the examination is repeated several times while the coitus-sampling interval is gradually reduced. Two or three examinations carried out 1 to 3 hours after sexual intercourse and showing consistently inconclusive or abnormal results are considered as clinically significant. The postcoital test, although a valuable indicator, may however not be sufficient to diagnose disturbed sperm/mucus interaction. In our clinics, a three-step approach has been developed for clinical screening of infertile couples to recognize and classify those in whom the main cause of infertility is inadequate sperm penetration. This method consists of the following elements:

1. cycle evaluation, including ovulation detection and timing, gross evaluation of cervical mucus properties, and postcoital tests (PCT)
2. seminal fluid analysis
3. evaluation of the cervical factor proper.

For evaluation of the physical properties and, by inference, of the chemical characteristics of the cervical mucus, a score of 12 points is used (Insler et al. 1970; Insler et al. 1972). This is a simple semiquantitative method of scoring up to 3 points for the amount, threadability, and crystallization capacity of the mucus as well as the degree of opening of the external cervical os. The total cervical score was empirically graded in four categories: negative, 0–3 points; initial, 4–7 points; good 8–10 points; and excellent, 11–12 points. Our group has shown that a good correlation existed between the cervical score and different ranges of total urinary estrogens (Fig. 8-4). Kerin et al. (1976) reported on an excellent correlation between the cervical score and the sperm penetrability of the mucus.

The first part of the three-step approach, i.e. the cycle evaluation, is of paramount importance, since it enables estimation of sperm/mucus interaction under hormonal conditions typical for the patient. It should be remembered that cervical mucus deficiency, with consequent impedance of sperm penetration, is frequently the result of anovulation and insufficient estrogen stimulation. In these cases, the cervical

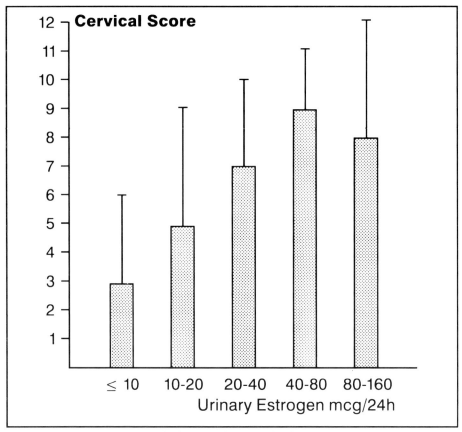

Fig. 8–4. Correlation between cervical score and estrogen levels.

factor, *per se,* could be normal. In addition to ovulation detection and mucus and PCT evaluation, the first step is also important for diagnosis of polyps, erosions, and displacements of the uterine cervix as well as inflammatory states of the lower genital tract. It is noteworthy, however, that these disturbances are rather rare in infertile patients.

The second step of the evaluation consists of seminal fluid analysis which includes measurement of the volume of the ejaculate, sperm count, evaluation of sperm motility and morphology, and estimation of fructose concentration (see Chapter 11: Semen analysis). When indicated, seminal fluid culture and split ejaculate analysis are carried out. Although labeled the second step, seminal fluid analysis is actually performed very early, simultaneously with the cycle evaluation.

The third part of the three-step approach includes the evaluation of the cervical factor proper (Insler, 1977). The aim of this procedure is to establish whether the patient's endocervical epithelium is capable of mucus production and, when produced, whether that mucus is of normal physical, chemical, and biological properties (sperm penetrabi-lity). The cervical crypts' ability to produce mucus is evaluated following stimulation with exogenous estrogen. The quality of mucus secreted is estimated by the cervical score. The response of the cervical crypts to estrogen is considered to be good when stimulation of the cervix results in a cervical score of 8 points or higher.

Biological properties of the mucus, i.e. its sperm penetrability, are estimated by in vitro sperm penetration tests using the method of Reichman et al. (1973a, 1973b). This technique enables calculation of the results in unequivocal quantitative terms. A microhematocrit tube filled with a mucus column 3 cm long is placed vertically in a drop of the semen to be tested. After incubation for 90 min, the tube with its mucus content is broken into three segments, each 1 cm long. Mucus from the upper segment is blown out into a slide, covered with a cover glass and examined under the microscope using a magnification of 400. The number of motile sperm cells is counted in at least ten microscopic fields. The results are expressed as the mean number of motile sperm per hpf, and subsequently graded as poor, inconclusive, or normal.

The sperm penetration test proposed by Kremer (1968) has also been frequently used for examination of the sperm mucus interaction. Practically, the evaluation of the cervical factor is performed as follows:

Patients are administered 75 micrograms (mcg) of ethinyl estradiol daily for 6–8 days beginning on the 5th day of spontaneous or induced bleeding. A mucus sample is collected on the 6th and 8th days of estrogen administration. The cervical score is estimated and a sperm penetration test is performed. The dose of ethinyl estradiol is then increased to 150 mcg per day for an additional 7–8 days and the same procedure of mucus sampling and sperm penetration tests is repeated. Following administration of estrogen alone for a total of 14–16 days, a combination of 75 mcg of ethinyl estradiol with 5 mg of medroxyprogesterone acetate is given for 5 days in order to provoke withdrawal bleeding.

The clinical evaluation of the cervical factor is performed by using the algorithmic approach shown in Figure 8–5.

If the initial seminal fluid analysis (SFA) is abnormal, the male partner's fertility potential must be evaluated and, if necessary, appropriately treated (see Chapter 11). If the SFA is normal and the female partner is able to produce adequate cervical mucus during a spontaneous menstrual cycle and the in vivo sperm penetration test, i.e. PCT, is normal, the sperm/mucus interaction may be considered to be adequate. Thus, at this stage, the cervical factor is diagnosed as normal.

If mucus production during the spontaneous cycle is insufficient, exogenous estrogens (EE) are administered according to the schedule described above. A failure of mucus production in response to a relatively high dose of estrogen may be diagnosed as cervical infertility or dysmucorrhea.

If administration of EE results in the production of adequate cervical mucus and the PCT is normal during the treated cycle, the problem of insufficient endogenous estrogen secretion should be considered. A repeated cycle evaluation also using estrogen assays and ultrasound observation of follicular development should be performed.

If, despite the fact that administration of EE resulted in production of physically normal mucus (score exceeding 8 points), the PCT is abnormal, the sperm/mucus interaction must be evaluated using the in vitro sperm penetration test (SP).

In cases with repeatedly negative PCT but showing a normal in vitro penetration test (SP), the problem is probably a disturbed sperm deposition.

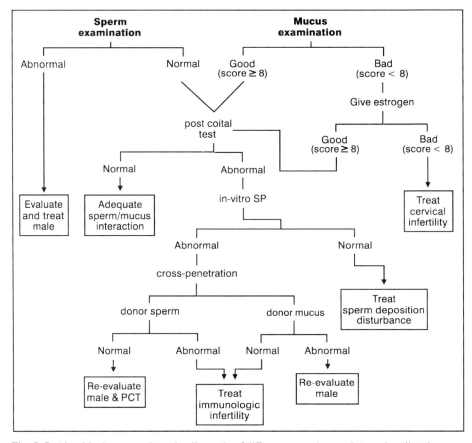

Fig. 8–5. Algorithmic approach to the diagnosis of different sperm/mucus interaction disturbances.

If both the PCT and the SP, i.e. the in vivo and in vitro sperm penetration, are abnormal, an in vitro cross-penetration test with donor mucus and sperm should be performed. Patients who produce cervical mucus hostile to sperm usually have abnormal in vitro penetration tests with both the husband's and donor sperm. The husband's sperm, however, readily penetrates donor mucus. In such cases the female partner's serum and cervical mucus should be examined for the presence of antisperm antibodies. If the tests are positive in both media (or only in the latter), the diagnosis of hostile mucus, i.e. immunological female infertility, may be established. The tests proposed for the detection of antisperm antibodies are numerous and express different basic approaches. The traditional sperm immobilization tests, the newer immunoperoxidase (IPAMA) assays, the sperm/cervical mucus contact test (SCMC), and the fashionable monoclonal antibodies techniques have been advocated and claimed to be superior to the others (Franklin & Dukes, 1964; Isojima et al. 1968; Friberg, 1974; Kremer et al. 1977; Holcberg et al. 1986; Hirschel et al. 1984; Isahakia & Alexander, 1984). However, the true incidence of antisperm

TABLE 8-1. Results of Cervical Factor Evaluation in 300 Infertile Couples. Since in several Couples the Evaluation was Repeated, the Total Number of Examinations was 342

Type of Disturbance	Number	%
Normal mucus & sperm penetr.	183	53.5
Relative dysmucorrhea	32	9.4
Absolute Dysmucorrhea	20	5.8
Penetration dysmucorrhea	25	7.3
Inherent sperm defect	82	24.0
Total	342	100.0

antibodies and their real meaning as a sole cause of female infertility still remain equivocal.

Using the three-step approach described above, 300 infertile couples were evaluated in 342 examinations. The results of this evaluation are summarized in Table 8-1. More than 62% of the examinations showed normal cervical factor and sperm. Complete inability of cervical mucus production was encountered in 5.8% of the women. It is of interest to note that none of these patients had undergone cervical surgery or extensive electrocoagulation, nor was cervical mucus infection frequent in the infertile female population examined. Of 156 cervical cultures, only 15 were contaminated with potentially pathogenic microorganisms. Moreover, the positive mucus cultures were spread at random throughout the whole population examined without any correlation whatsoever to a specific cervical pathology. Hostile cervical mucus, i.e. possibly immunological infertility, was detected in 7.3% of the cases. The frequency of cervical mucus hostility is somewhat lower in our material than the incidence of antisperm antibodies found by various authors in the female partners of infertile couples (Shulman, 1972; Mettler & Shirvani, 1975).

One additional finding of this series should be noted. Inherent sperm defect, indicated by normal penetration of the wife's mucus by donor sperm and reduced penetrating ability of the husband's spermatozoa through both the wife's and donor mucus, was found in 82 out of 342 examinations (24%). In 56 of these men, the seminal fluid analysis was performed within 60 days of the cervical factor evaluation. Judging by sperm count, motility, and morphology, 50%, 77% and 71% of these males respectively would be considered fertile. However, only in 10 patients (18%), were all three seminal fluid parameters normal and, in 48%, two or three parameters (count, motility, or morphology) were definitely abnormal. In all these patients, sperm penetration through the wife's and donor mucus was significantly reduced. This indicates an inherent biological deficiency of the spermatozoa. Such a deficiency could not be detected by the routine seminal fluid analysis in 10 of the 56 males examined. It seems that the in vitro sperm penetration test may also serve as an important tool in the evaluation of male fertility potential (Insler et al. 1979).

TREATMENT OF INFERTILITY DUE TO THE CERVICAL FACTOR

The general approach to classification and treatment of infertility due to disturbed cervical function may be summarized as follows:

In cases of reduced sperm penetration due to estrogen deficiency, the evaluation of the cervical factor reveals a normal response of the endocervical mucosa to exogenous stimulation. Following the administration of ethinyl estradiol, abundant mucus of normal physical and biological qualities is produced. In these cases the cervical factor, *per se,* is normal and induction of ovulation with clomiphene citrate or with human gonadotropins will result in proper stimulation of the cervix, production of adequate mucus, and normal sperm penetration.

Persistently bad postcoital tests, concomitant with reduced penetration of the husband's sperm through both the wife's and donor mucus, indicate an inherent sperm defect which may or may not be evident in seminal fluid examination.

In cases with abnormal postcoital tests repeatedly showing a complete absence of sperm in the cervical mucus but producing a good cervical mucus readily penetrable by the husband's sperm in vitro, the main problem is disturbed sperm deposition. In extremely rare and readily diagnosed cases, the disturbed sperm deposition may be due to anatomical reasons such as different degrees of hypospadias, cervical displacement, or severe uterine prolapse. The vast majority of cases, however, result from impeded sexual function. Faulty coital technique or hidden or unreported impotence are the main reasons for this disturbance. In such cases, artificial insemination with the husband's sperm is the most efficient treatment. It must be remembered that this therapy is merely an effective medical solution and should never be applied without a concomitant psychological and/or behavioral sex therapy.

Failure of the endocervical crypts to react to estrogen stimulation (dysmucorrhea) may be a late sequele to an inflammatory process or a consequence of surgical procedures such as conization, amputation, or electrocoagulation of the uterine cervix. However, there have to be other causes still unknown, since in our material none of the patients had cervical surgery and virtually all had sterile cervical mucus cultures.

Treatment of dysmucorrhea is still a rather vague proposition. It is actually not known whether damaged cervical secretory units are at all capable of regeneration and re-establishment of normal function. The application of antibiotics and hormones (Marcus & Marcus, 1968; Elstein, 1974) and stimulation of the endocervical epithelium by electrocoagulation (Marcus & Marcus, 1968) or by cervical curettage (our own unpublished results) has proven to be ineffective. More recently, it has been shown that cervical infertility can be successfully treated by intrauterine insemination using either split ejaculate or washed husband's sperm (Glezerman & Jecht, 1984). GIFT or IVF may also be considered (Hewitt et al. 1985).

The treatment of cervical mucus hostility, i.e. the immunological incompatibility between spermatozoa and cervical secretion, is still a controversial subject. Shulman proposed a high-dosage corticosteroids therapy (Shulman & Shulman, 1982). Other authors reported encouraging results using intrauterine insemination (Glezerman & Jecht, 1984; Kerin et al. 1984; Sher et al. 1984). Condom-protected sexual intercourse was advocated by several authors (Franklin & Dukes, 1964; Behrman, 1968) but has produced contradictory results. Recently IVF has been suggested as an efficient treatment of immunologic infertility (Navot & Schenker, 1985; De Almeida et al. 1987). Our preliminary results seem to indicate that IVF using cord serum instead of the patient's serum and carefully cleaning the ova of the surrounding cumulus cells before adding spermatozoa to the culture wells may improve the results of IVF treatment in women with antisperm antibodies.

The exact mechanism of the production of cervical mucus has not yet been fully revealed. Many details of sperm/mucus interaction are still obscure and the information on immunological causes of infertility is as confusing as it is voluminous. Hence, the diagnosis, classification, and treatment of cervical diseases leading to infertility are still preliminary and empirical. Until a comprehensive classification of cervical malfunctions is developed and generally adopted, effective therapy of these disturbances cannot be designed.

Male Infertility

9. MALE INFERTILITY PROCESSES

PHYSIOLOGY OF TESTICULAR FUNCTION

The testes fulfill two tasks: steroidogenesis, a process that takes place in the Leydig (interstitial) cells, situated between the seminiferous tubules; and spermatogenesis, which takes place in the germinal epithelium of these tubules. The germ cells undergo six developmental stages before spermatozoa reach maturation. These changes comprise 3 phases: 1) proliferation of spermatogonia, 2) reduction divisions (meioses), and 3) spermiogenesis, i.e. the metamorphosis of spermatids into spermatozoa. In many species, including man, testicular sperm are incapable of fertilizing the ovum. During the passage through the epididymis, however, they become functionally mature and capable of fertilization. Both the acquisition of fertilizing ability and the maintenance of the structural and functional integrity of the epididymis are dependent upon the presence of androgens.

The regulation of testicular function is governed by an interplay between the hypothalamus, hypophysis, and the testes (Fig. 9-1). The hypothalamic-pituitary-testicular axis may be defined, in simplified terms, as a system following cybernetic rules. In such an analogy, the role of the command circuit is performed by the hypothalamus (GnRH). The role of the regulating circuit is played by the pituitary gland (FSH, LH). Testicular secretions such as sex steroids and inhibin, on the other hand, assume the function of modulators issuing feedback signals. Any disruption of this system or dysfunction of its components may lead to infertility. The components of this system, the regulation of this functional circuit, and the effects of its disruption are the essential topics of this chapter.

The Hypothalamus-Pituitary Axis

Topographic and functional aspects of the hypothalamus-pituitary axis have been dealt with elsewhere in this book. The hormones involved, namely gonadotropin-releasing hormone (GnRH) and gonadotropins (FSH and LH), are identical for both male and female and have been discussed in earlier sections of this book.

For many years it was believed that the hypothalamus-pituitary axis functions substantially differently in males and females.

This assumption was based on the observation of the dramatic changes in gonadotropin and steroid secretions in the course of the female menstrual cycle as opposed to the continuous nature of sperm production and the relative uniformity of gonadotropin and steroid secretion in the male. Today, there is no doubt that GnRH and gonadotropins are secreted in both male and female in a pulsatile fashion (Santen & Bardin, 1973; Carmel et al. 1976). Long-term changes in gonadotropin levels, such as those observed during the female menstrual cycle, are a result of modulations by gonadal products (steroids, inhibin) and do indeed differ between men and women. Knobil (1980) and Knobil et al. (1980) have shown in their classical study that abolition of the pulsatile pattern of GnRH secretion causes severe gonadal dysfunction in both females and males.

The pulsatile nature of GnRH and gonadotropin secretion should not have come as a total surprise. All biological functions are endowed with a rhythmic pattern.

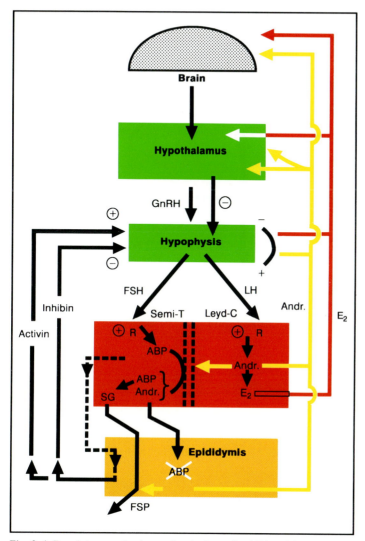

Fig. 9-1. Regulatory mechanisms of testicular and epididymal function. For explanation see p. 122; Semi-T = seminiferous tubules; Leyd-C = Leydig cells; R = receptor; Andr. = androgen; ABP = androgen binding protein; SG = spermatogenesis; FSP = presumably fertile spermatozoa.

These may range from several Hertz to daily or seasonal variations. Pulses may be dependent on the sleep/wake rhythm, like the secretion of prolactin, or may be dependent on an inherent central rhythm, as with cortisol. Yet, it is not the target organ which is dependent on rhythmic stimulation. Both ovarian and testicular function have been successfully restored by uniform doses of gonadotropins. However, pulsatile gonadal stimulation with normal frequency and amplitude of pulses optimizes or at least improves testicular function (Wagner et al. 1985).

Current view regards the four basic components of the testis, namely Sertoli cells, Leydig cells, germ cells and peritubular cells, as a closely interdependent unit which is controlled by autocrine, paracrine and endocrine actions (Fig. 9-2). For an extensive

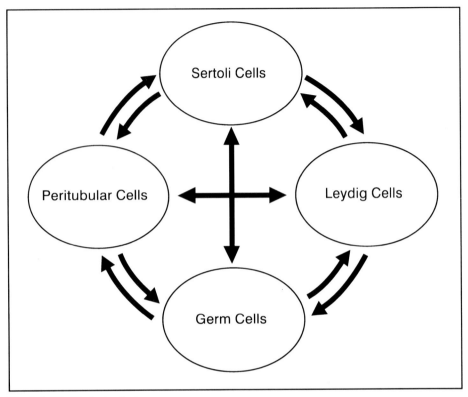

Fig. 9-2. The Testicular System.

discussion see the excellent reviews by Heindel and Treinen (1989) and Skinner (1991).

The Sertoli Cell (SC)

Over 120 years ago, Sertoli described a distinct cell type within the seminiferous tubules which line the peritubular membrane and extend towards the tubular lumen (Sertoli, 1865). Like nerve cells, these cells proliferate only during fetal and perinatal life. Many roles have been attributed to the Sertoli cell, such as being a structural support for the tubules and a nursing cell. But the central role of the Sertoli cell in the control of spermatogenesis has been fully appreciated only in recent years. Spermatogenesis takes place within folds of the cytoplasm of the SC. Tight junctions between adjacent SCs divide the spermatogenetic line into an adluminal and a basal compartment and impede the diffusion of materials from the interstitial space into the seminiferous tubules. It is this complex of tight junctions which form the blood – testes barrier. The SC is capable of steroidogenesis, the specific activity being 40–140 times lower than that observed in the Leydig cells (Christensen and Mason, 1976). Furthermore the SC produces a variety of macromolecules such as androgen-binding protein (ABP), plasminogen activators, transferrin, the anti-Muellerian hormone, and a substance with GnRH-like activity (Steinberger, 1986). The Sertoli cell also plays a role in the regulation of Leydig cells. Verhoeven and Caileau (1985) have noted a factor in spent media from rat SCs that stimulates steroidogenesis by Leydig cells in vitro. Buch et al. (1988) have detected a growth factor in conditioned media from rat and human SCs with unique physiochemical properties, distinct from other known growth factors. This factor, termed by the authors „Sertoli cell secreted growth factor" may play a key role in normal spermatogenesis or in Leydig cell function.

Steroidogenesis of Leydig cells is probably modulated by a variety of products derived from Sertoli cells: IGF-1 (Lin et al. 1986), TGF-B (Skinner and Moses, 1989) seem to increase steroidogenesis while IL-1 (Calkins et al. 1988) among others decrease steroidogenesis by Leydig cells.

Even the size of Leydig cells may be controlled to an extent by secretions of Sertoli cells such as TGF-a (Skinner et al. 1989).

The Sertoli cell is the main (Steinberger et al. 1975; Santiemma et al. 1984) but not the exclusive (Orth & Christensen, 1978) target cell for FSH in the rat and in the human.

It is established that FSH binds at specific membrane receptors on the Sertoli cells and activates adenyl cyclase. Cyclic AMP, formed in response to this stimulus, promotes DNA-dependent RNA synthesis resulting in the formation of androgen receptors and the synthesis of androgen-binding protein (ABP) (Walsh et al. 1970; Louis et al. 1975; Steinberger et al. 1975). Spermatogenesis may, at least in some species, be initiated without FSH. This has been confirmed in vivo: it has been shown that mice whose endogenous gonadotropin production was suppressed from birth by anti-rat gonadotropin serum had the same testicular development as untreated controls during the first week of life. In the second week of life, spermatocytes were found in testicular preparations of controls as well as of treated animals, although in the latter, the number of spermatocytes and spermatogonia were reduced. None of the animals kept free of gonadotropin was capable of forming spermatids but administration of FSH led to a testicular picture resembling that of the controls (Lunenfeld and Weissenberg, 1972). The ABP-androgen complex within the cytoplasm of the Sertoli cell provides a reservoir for androgens in the seminiferous tubules from which androgens can be drawn to stimulate spermatogenesis.

The Leydig Cell (LC)

The Leydig cells, first described by Leydig in 1850, are epithelial polygonal cells with a prominent nucleus and abundant endoplasmatic reticulum. The LCs undergo two phases of development, the first during the fetal life and the second during puberty. They develop as early as in the 8th week of fetal life. At the end of the 14th week of pregnancy, some 50% of the mass of the testes are composed of Leydig cells. (For comparison, the LC in the adult testes form only some 10% of the total mass of the testes.) The fetal LCs secrete testosterone, and the peripheral testosterone in the 14–18 weeks old fetus is within the adult range. In the second part of fetal life, the number of LCs diminishes continuously, but they are still detectable at birth. At about six months after birth, the testes are virtually void of LCs. Under LH stimulation during puberty, LCs are again formed from fibroblasts.

LCs are the main target for LH. LH molecules bind to specific, high-affinity, low-capacity receptors in the interstitial Leydig cells (Dufau et al. 1973; Major & Kilpatrick, 1972; Moudgal et al. 1971; Moyle et al. 1971) and induce the conversion of cholesterol to androgens, which are the main product of the Leydig cells. Leydig cells also secrete oxytocin which is thought to cause contraction of myoid cells surrounding the seminiferous tubules (Sharpe, 1988). Furthermore, Pro-Opio-Melano-Cortin is secreted by Leydig cells and the various peptides derived from this substance may serve as paracrine regulators of Sertoli cell function (Bardin et al. 1984).

In the adult, approximately 7 mg of testosterone are produced daily (Lipsett, 1971). FSH may also play a role in regulating LC function. It has been shown in vivo that FSH administration to immature hypophysectomized rats was followed by an increase in LH receptors and steroidogenesis (Chen et al. 1976; Selin & Moger, 1977).

Peritubular Cells

Peritubular cells are contractible myoid cells which surround the seminiferous tubules. They contain androgen and oxytocin receptors and are therefore, to an extent, regulated by Leydig cells. There seems to exist a very intricate system of paracrine cooperation between peritubular cells and Sertoli cells: Both produce different "raw materials" to the formation of the tubular wall (Tung and Fritz, 1980). Co-cultures of Sertoli cells and peritubular cells survive significantly longer than each cell type in monoculture (Hutson and Stocco, 1981). Skinner and Fritz (1985) have isolated from peritubular cell cultures a factor, which has been termed "P-mod-S" (Peritubular modulator of Sertoli cells). As implicated by the name, this substance modulates secretions of Sertoli cells.

Androgens and Estrogens

Intratesticular androgens diffuse into the Sertoli cells, are bound to ABP, and subsequently released for stimulation of spermatogenesis (Lacy, 1972, 1974; Setchell, 1976; Van Der Molen et al. 1972). In addition, androgens stimulate the development of the accessory glands, promote the development of secondary sex characteristics, exert metabolic and psychic effects, and finally participate in the complex feedback mechanism that ensures appropriate gonadotropin secretion.

Androgen receptors have also been demonstrated on Sertoli cells (Nakhla et al. 1984; Isomaa et al. 1985). Marshall and Nieschlag (1987) have concluded that many of the effects of FSH on the Sertoli cells can also be achieved by androgen action on these cells, albeit through a different mechanism.

Cessation of testicular secretion by gonadectomy is followed by an increase in GnRH activity in the hypophyseal portal blood and, consequently, by an elevation of gonadotropin levels (Ben-Jonathan et al. 1973). Furthermore, Mogulewsky et al. (1974) demonstrated that incubation of labeled tyrosine with hypothalamic slices from castrated rats produced significantly more biologically active GnRH than comparable slices from normal rats. Adding testosterone to the incubation medium inhibited the synthesis of GnRH. Since the hypothalamus contains enzymes which aromatize androgens (Martini et al. 1974; Naftolin et al. 1972), it cannot be excluded that the inhibitory effect was due, at least in part, to testosterone conversion into estrogens.

TABLE 9-1. Hormonal Profile of a castrated Patient before and following Administration of Testosterone Propionate (TP; 25 mg/day for 3 days) and Mesterolone (M; 75 mg/day for 3 weeks)*

	Before	After TP	After M
FSH mIU	27.0	0.8	18.25
LH mIU	15.3	1.0	21.0
T NG	2.0	12.0	1.3
E2 pg	> 20.0	52.5	> 20.0

* Each hormone level indicated in the Table represents a mean value.
Individual FSH and LH levels are shown in Table 9-2.

Estrogens were also shown to strongly inhibit gonadotropic release (Eldridge et al. 1974). On the other hand, neither dihydrotestosterone nor mesterolone – saturated derivatives of testosterone which usually are not aromatized to estrogens (Braun and Sepsenwol, 1974) – are capable of inhibiting gonadotropins (Laschet and Laschet, 1966, 1968). The above evidence seems to indicate that it is estrogen or a combination of estrogen and testosterone rather than testosterone alone which exerts the feedback action upon the hypothalamus and the pituitary. This hypothesis is strengthened by the following clinical example: A castrated male with elevated FSH and LH levels and low plasma testosterone and estradiol was given testosterone propionate (25 mg/day) and subsequently mesterolone (75 mg/day). Following the administration of testosterone propionate, FSH and LH levels decreased significantly within 3 days, while both testosterone and estradiol showed a significant rise, indicating that a part of the exogenous testosterone propionate was aromatized and converted into estrogen. In contrast, the administration of mesterolone for 3 consecutive weeks failed to influence either the estrogen or the gonadotropin levels. Concomitant administration of GnRH and testosterone propionate resulted in an increased gonadotropin release, while mesterolone did not enhance the pituitary response to GnRH (Tables 9-1, 9-2). This example shows that the inhibitory feedback effect of steroids is exerted mainly at the hypothalamic level by estrogen rather than by androgens.

TABLE 9-2. Response to GnRH in a castrated Patient before and following administration of Testosterone Propionate (TP; 25 mg/day for 3 days) and mesterolone (M; 75 mg/day for 3 weeks)

	Before		After TP		After M	
Min.	FSH (mIU)	LH (mIU)	FSH (mIU)	LH (mIU)	FSH (mIU)	LH (mIU)
- 10	33.0	13.3	0.9	0.5	18.8	21.0
0	24.0	17.3	0.7	1.5	18.8	21.5
30	27.7	39.0	2.0	3.2	23.8	38.0
60		40.0	2.4	7.2	30.8	117.0
120	36.7	23.0	3.7	12.8	26.2	62.0
180	27.7	14.8	10.2	28.0	33.0	25.5

TABLE 9-3. Response to GnRH (100 μg) before and during Cyproterone Acetate

	Control		Response during Cyproterone Acetate	
Time	LH mIU/ml	FSH mIU/ml	LH mIU/ml	FSH mUI/ml
Control 1	–	< 0.5	2.2	2.5
Control 2	3.4	< 0.5	2.2	2.8
10'	–	–	6.3	1.9
30'	23.5	2.5	6.2	2.2
60'	19.8	2.6	6.0	–
90'	–	–	4.0	2.6
120'	9.1	2.5	3.8	3.15
180'	9.9	2.4	3.8	2.5

We have shown that the anti-androgen, cyproterone acetate, decreased pituitary responsiveness to GnRH with respect to both FSH and LH release (Table 9-3).

Steroid regulation of gonadotropic secretion may also be modulated by virtue of testosterone-estradiol-binding globulin's capacity to alter the level of free sex steroids. Furthermore, changes in the levels or activity of steroid-metabolizing enzymes within the hypothalamus or pituitary may also be important in regulating gonadotropic secretion.

Inhibin

As an additional mechanism controlling the secretion of FSH, the seminiferous tubules secrete inhibin, a substance specifically inhibiting FSH release (Franchimont, 1972, 1973a; Johnson, 1970, 1972; Bandivdekar et al. 1982). Suggestive evidence comes from clinical conditions involving selective dysfunction of the seminiferous tubules. This is well illustrated in patients with Sertoli-cell-only syndrome who exhibit elevated FSH titers concomitant with normal LH and testosterone levels (Table 9-4).

Since inhibin acts by modulating pituitary responsiveness, lack of inhibin in these patients is expressed as exaggerated FSH and normal LH response to GnRH stimulation. A similar hormonal profile in patients with Klinefelter's syndrome

TABLE 9-4. A Patient with Sertoli-Cell-Only Syndrome, exhibiting high FSH titer but normal LH, Testosterone and estradiol titers. Dynamic test using GnRH shows exaggerated FSH response contrasted to a normal LH response

FSH mIU	LH mIU	Testosterone ng	E_2 pg	Min.
22	3.9			–20
23	4.2	9.6	20	0
48				15
65	8.8			30
56				60
96	9.9			90
158				150
62	5.5	12.8		180

TABLE 9-5. Plasma Follicle Stimulating Hormone (FSH) and Luteinizing Hormone (LH) Concentratios in male castrated Rats injected daily for 5 days with Saline, rete Testis Fluid (RTF) or Testosterone Propionate (TP). Modified from Setchell and Jacks, 1974

Exp.	FSH ng/ml	%	LH RP-1/ml	%
Saline	2200	100	10.5	100
RTF	1207	55	10.5	100
TP	1260	57	2.0	19

(Bonati, 1974) corroborates this evidence. In the absence of spermatogenesis, and thus in the absence of inhibin, FSH levels (both basal and following GnRH stimulation) are disproportionately high.

Inhibin is produced and secreted by the Sertoli cells (Steinberger and Steinberger, 1976; Bicsak et al. 1987). It has been shown by Setchell and Jacks (1974) that, whereas testosterone propionate injected into castrated rats reduced both FSH and LH levels, RTF from fertile rams significantly reduced FSH without influencing LH levels (Table 9-5). The selective inhibition of FSH secretion by RTF suggested a direct effect on the pituitary. A substance with inhibin-like activity has been isolated from testes fluid (Setchell, 1974a, 1974b) and has also been isolated and characterized from pooled seminal fluid (Ramasharma et al. 1984). Its complete amino sequence has been reported by Seidah et al. (1984). A preparation believed to have a purity in the range of 10 – 30% has been presented by Rivier et al. (1986).

Inhibins represent a group of substances rather than a single hormone. Inhibins may originate from multiple sites and may have multiple actions within the reproductive system (Moodbidri et al. 1987). Leydig cells may also be a source of inhibin. Roberts et al. (1989) have reported inhibin immuno-staining and subunit mRNAs in fixed Leydig cells of the rat. Risbridger et al. (1989) have confirmed this observation in cultured rat cells. Consequently, LH and hCG increase circulating inhibin levels in men with testosterone-induced gonadotropin suppression (McLachlan, 1988). Winters (1989) has observed coinciding testosterone and inhibin pulses in the spermatic vein. He concluded that the same mechanism responsible for the release of testosterone from the testes also stimulates inhibin release. Chappel (1987) has compiled literature on the origins of inhibins (Table 9-6).

TABLE 9-6. Tissues that contain nonsteroidal FSH Inhibitory Activity (modified from Chappel, 1987)

Male	Female
Rete testis fluid	Follicular fluid
Testicular tissue	Ovarian venous blood
Sperm extracts	Ovarian extracts
Seminal plasma	Granulosa cell culture
Testicular lymph	
Sertoli cell culture	
Peripheral blood	

Inhibin is a heterodimer composed of an alpha and a beta subunit. The latter is actually formed of two subunits (A and B). Beta subunits may recombine as homodimers (A+A) or heterodimers (A+B). These substances are termed Activin A (homodimer) and Activin B (heterodimer). While inhibin inhibits the release of FSH secretion but not LH secretion, both activins are specific in exclusively stimulating the secretion of FSH (Vale et al. 1986; Ling et al. 1986). In human seminal plasma, at least three molecular variants of inhibin have been described, ranging from 1,500 to 10,400 daltons (Arbatti and Sheth, 1987). The common biological properties of all of these is the selective inhibition of FSH release by the pituitary gland. However, inhibin may also act on the hypothalamic level, reducing the synthesis of GnRH (Moodbidri et al. 1981), and may affect the gonads by interfering with FSH binding to gonadal receptors (Bandivdekar et al. 1984). At present it is not clear whether the variety of actions attributed to the inhibins may be due to contaminants or to breakdown products of inhibin. The currently accepted view defines inhibin as a nonsteroid hormone produced by the seminiferous tubules under FSH control and in the presence of intact spermatogenesis. It regulates the synthesis and basal secretion of FSH and modulates the pituitary response to GnRH as far as FSH secretion is concerned.

Further research on inhibins will undoubtedly improve our insight into the physiology of human reproduction. The availability of sensitive and specific radio-immuno-assays (Arbatti and Sheth, 1987) will pave the way.

Prolactin

A mounting body of evidence suggests a role for prolactin (PRL) in the male reproductive organs. Binding sites for PRL have been identified on Leydig cells (Charreau et al. 1977). A synergistic effect of PRL with circulating androgens has been demonstrated and a stimulatory effect of PRL on androgen production has been shown both in testes and the adrenals (Negro-Vilar, 1980). PRL seems also to directly affect spermatogenesis by interfering with spermatid differentiation (Sheriff, 1984). Thus, elevated PRL levels may be associated with an increase in abnormally configurated spermatozoa in the ejaculate (Toth, 1981). Laufer et al. (1981) and Perryman and Thorner (1981) have reported on oligozoospermia associated with hyperprolactinemia. Del Pozo (1982) has compiled frequencies of clinical symptoms and signs in male hyperprolactinemia from the literature (Table 9-7).

TABLE 9-7. Incidence of Symptoms of Hyperprolactinemia in Men
(after Del Pozo, 1982)

Signs	Incidence (%)
Impotence	80
Hypoandrogenism and hypospermatogenesis	65
Visual impairment	61
Headache	27
Gynecomastia	9.5
Galactorrhea	3

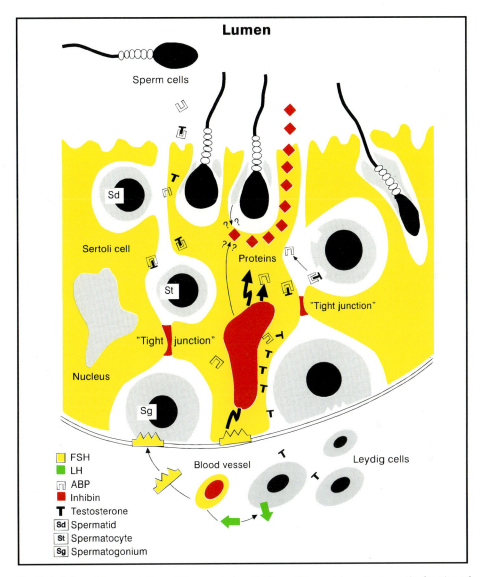

Fig. 9–3. Schematic presentation of the germinal epithelium with special emphasis on the function of Sertoli cells in the regulation of spermatogenesis (see text). From: Lunenfeld and Glezerman, 1981.

Spermatogenesis

The process that produces mature and motile sperm cells can be divided into three phases. The first phase is called spermatogenesis. This phase is basically the development of haploid spermatids from diploid spermatogonia. The resulting round spermatids, which still do not resemble sperm cells, have to undergo further differentiation. This process, which includes the formation of the acrosome, the tail, condensation of the nucleus, and the eventual loss of the cytoplasmatic body, is the second phase in the development of the mature sperm cell. At the end of this phase, termed spermiogenesis, the sperm cell is released into the lumen of the seminiferous tubule and has all the morphological features of mature spermatozoa. Heller and Clermont (1964) have calculated that the first two phases require 74 + 6 days to complete. Yet, after having undergone these two phases, the sperm cells are still not capable of fertilization. A further step of maturation is required. This third phase, the maturation phase, occurs in the epididymis after the release of the spermatozoa from the seminiferous tubules. During the passage of the spermatozoa from the head of the epididymis through the body and the tail of this organ, the spermatozoa undergo further morphological, biochemical, and metabolic changes which provide the cells with their fertilizing potential. These changes include an increase in the content of cyclic AMP and an increase of the specific weight and the oxygen consumption rate. The journey of the sperm cells through the epididymis takes 1–21 days with a mean of 12 days (Rowley et al. 1970). As a result of this rather prolonged transit time, the epididymis also acts as a storage space for mature sperm cells.

Spermatogenesis and spermiogenesis take place within cytoplasmatic folds of the Sertoli cells (Fig. 9–3). The intimate proximity of maturing sperm cells to the cytoplasm of the Sertoli cells forms the ideal topographic basis for metabolic exchange. The Sertoli cell is the only cell within the seminiferous tubule which borders both, at the tubular membrane and the tubular lumen. Various substances, such as inhibin, produced during spermiogenesis, is able to leave the tubule through the cytoplasm of the Sertoli cells, and substrates originating in the interstitium find access to the maturing sperm cells via the cytoplasm of the Sertoli cell. Of particular importance is the access of androgens to the maturing sperm cells. Androgens are produced by interstitial Leydig cells. Diffusion of any material across spaces between Sertoli cells is possible only up to the so-called tight junctions, which are formed by the membranes of adjacent Sertoli cells (Dym and Fawcett, 1970; Fawcett, 1975). These tight junctions form the blood-testes barrier. Substrates derived from blood vessels in the interstitium or excreted from the Leydig cells therefore have to pass the cytoplasm of the Sertoli cell in order to reach maturing sperm cells. A simple diffusion process would not suffice to create the high concentrations required. Some form of an active transport mechanism within the cytoplasm of the SC is necessary. Steinberger (1977) has stated that the processes of spermatogenesis and spermiogenesis require the androgen concentration within the tubular epithelium to be 100 times higher than the peripheral concentration. The mechanism by which this extremely high intratubular concentration is achieved depends on the production of an androgen-binding protein (ABP) by the Sertoli cell. ABP, which has a high affinity to androgen, traps diffused testosterone and the ABP-testosterone complex moves within the cytoplasm of the SC to the folds which contain the maturing sperm cells. Nuclear receptors for androgens have been demonstrated in these cells (Sanborn et al. 1975; Wright and Frenkel, 1980; Isomaa et al. 1985). Androgens are released from the ABP-androgen complex and bind to these receptors. Androgens are the principal stimulators of spermatogenesis and spermiogenesis and the Sertoli cell , which produces ABP under the influence of FSH, enables the required high androgen concentrations to reach the maturing sperm cells. The mechanism by which the seminiferous tubules exert a negative feedback on the pituitary and regulate FSH secretion depends on the production of inhibin. This substance leaves the tubules via the cytoplasm of the SC and gains access to the vascular system in the interstitium.

On the basis of the above facts, it can be postulated that the control and coordination of testicular function (seminiferous tubules and Leydig cells) is accomplished by 3 types of actions (Fig. 9-1):

1. Stimulations along the brain-hypothalamus-hypophysis-testes axis by GnRH and gonadotropins.
2. Intratesticular modulation consisting of the activation of appropriate hormone receptors (R) and dynamic changes of inhibin, activin and steroid concentrations. FSH, after binding to membrane receptors, activates adenyl cyclase. Cyclic AMP formed in response to this stimulus promotes DNA-dependent RNA synthesis resulting in the formation of inhibin, ABP, and probably aromatase and 5-alpha reductase in the seminiferous tubules. LH stimulates production of androgens by the Leydig cells. Testosterone reaches the proper concentration within the seminiferous tubules by the ABP transport mechanism and is there partly reduced to dehydrotestosterone (DHT) and partly converted to E-2. Androgen within the seminiferous tubules then stimulates spermatogenesis. Some of the ABP-androgen complexes reach the epididymis together with sperm containing testicular fluid. Proteinase in the epididymis digest the ABP, thus creating a high concentration of free androgen. This is probably necessary to maintain the structural and functional integrity of the epididymis and for the acquisition of fertilizing ability by the spermatozoa.
3. Feedback signals, positive (+) and negative (-), exerted by testicular steroids and inhibin:
   a) testicular steroids inhibit hypothalamic GnRH secretion
   b) androgens diminish pituitary responsiveness to GnRH with respect to LH release, but have no significant effect on FSH
   c) estrogens potentiate LH secretion in response to GnRH
   d) testicular inhibin reduces and activin increases FSH secretion by modulating pituitary responsiveness to GnRH
   e) changes in the levels or activity of steroid-metabolizing enzymes within the hypothalamus or pituitary also play a role in the regulation of gonadotropic secretion.

Any disruption of the delicately coordinated interaction between the components of the hypothalamic-pituitary-testicular axis may lead to infertility.

ERECTION AND EJACULATION

The reproductive competence of the male requires adequate sexual function. The parapendymal tract transmits neural impulses from the infundibular nucleus on the floor of the third ventricle via the spinal cord to the sacral plexus, which controls erection and ejaculation sequences.

Erection, the result of tumescence of the penile cavernous bodies, is mediated by parasympathetic impulses passing through the nervi erigentes from the second to the fourth sacral cord segments. Sympathetic nerve fibers from higher levels may also transmit impulses via the hypogastric plexus, resulting in erection. These nerve fibers as well as the parasympathetic ones concerned with erection are cholinergic.

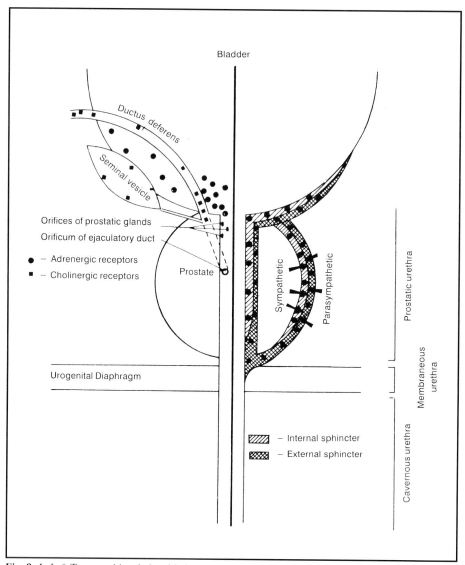

Fig. 9–4. *Left:* Topographic relationship between the ductus deferens, seminal vesicle, and prostate and their outlets into the prostatic urethra. Note the dense adrenergic innervation of the bladder neck and cholinergic innervation of the ductus deferens and the seminal vesicle.
Right: Topographic scheme of the internal and external sphincters. Whether the external sphincter really enters the capsule of the prostate has not been fully elucidated to date. (Glezerman et al., 1976 b)

Ejaculation is a reflex action and can be divided into two stages (Masters & Johnson, 1966). During the first stage, the emission (Rieser, 1961), sperm cells from the epididymis and seminal fluid from the prostate and the seminal vesicle are pumped into the posterior urethra by active contractions of the epididymis, the ductus deferens, and the seminal vesicles. Due to a delicate synchronization mechanism, the contributions of the epididymis, the prostate, and the seminal vesicles are expelled successively.

Fractionated ejaculation and the detection of specific markers in the different portions enable the detection of synchronization failures. The first stage of the ejaculating process seems to be under parasympathetic control (Retieff, 1950; Potts, 1957). Concomitantly with the arrival of the seminal fluid into the prostatic part of the urethra, the bladder neck is closed by contraction of the internal urethral sphincter. This prevents the sperm from being ejected backwards into the bladder. The very dense sympathetic innervation of the bladder neck is thought to play an important role in the closing of the bladder neck (Fig. 9–4). It seems that the arrival of the semen in the prostatic part of the urethra triggers the second stage of ejaculation. Afferent impulses excite the sacral and lumbar cord (Retieff, 1950), which then discharge impulses over autonomous and sympathetic pathways, resulting in rhythmic contractions of the ischiocavernosus and bulbocavernosus muscles as well as the perineal muscles. Thus, the semen is forcefully propelled via the urethra through the external meatus while the external sphincter urethrae relaxes. Relaxation of this sphincter seems to be under parasympathetic control.

It appears that the ejaculatory process is a rather complex phenomenon involving simultaneous and subsequent sympathetic and parasympathetic stimulation of different organs and structures in the male genital tract.

10. DIAGNOSIS OF MALE INFERTILITY

HISTORY

A general history of the couple will provide information about the age of the partners, duration of marriage, duration of unprotected coitus, previous use of contraceptive methods, whether there is adequate knowledge and use of the fertile period, past fertility of each of the partners during the present or previous unions, results of investigations already performed by other physicians, and previous or current treatment for infertility. Any diseases, treatments, or surgery which might potentially influence fertility should be recorded. For example: clamping or tearing of the vas deferens in very young patients undergoing repair of bilateral cryptorchidism or congenital hernia is the most frequent traumatic cause of obstruction.

Since certain familiar diseases may affect fertility, it is essential that information concerning some typical diseases be recorded (e.g. diabetes mellitus, thyroid disorders, tuberculosis, hypertension, vascular diseases, DES exposure).

The history of past illness should be as complete as possible and should include trivial long-standing infections and childhood illnesses. Alterations in spermatogenesis may be brought about by apparently harmless illnesses, such as measles and simple pneumonia, as well as by serious infections such as typhoid. One should especially search for diseases such as syphilis, gonorrhea, mycoplasma, chlamydia, and nonspecific urethritis, since these or their sequels may adversely affect fertility. The deleterious influence of raised temperature and protracted febrile illness on spermatogenesis is well-known and may lead to oligozoospermia, asthenospermia, or teratospermia. Any febrile disease or acute incident during a six-month period preceding a semen analysis could result in a temporary decrease of quantity and quality of sperm. The age factor needs to be taken into consideration in the history. Prepubertal mumps orchitis is frequently benign and runs a reversible course. However, after puberty it may cause irreversible damage. Febrile or toxic damage to the spermatogenic system also seems to occur more frequently after puberty.

It should be ascertained whether both testes have always been in the scrotum. If not, the type of treatment given to correct this condition should be noted. If there was a history of bilateral cryptorchidism in the past, fertility prognosis is extremely poor, independent of the age at which surgery was performed. This must be differentiated from mobile testis or conditions in which the descent of testis was obtained by medical treatment alone. In this case prognosis is better. A corrected unilateral cryptorchidism may have a good fertility prognosis. Injury to the testes, epididymitis-orchitis, and urinary disease may all be potential causes of a fertility problem. Torsion of testis, especially when diagnosis and detorsion were delayed, may lead to atrophy and impaired fertility. However, patients who were operated on not more than 8 hours after the onset of symptoms have been found to have normally-sized testicles and only slight changes in testicular morphology and sperm parameters. Thus, when medical history reveals past testicular torsion, the time element should be thoroughly investigated. Excessive consumption of alcohol (more than 60 g per day), tobacco, narcotics, or regular use of hot baths or sauna may also lead to temporary infertility.

It has been reported that some types of respiratory diseases are associated with infertility: patients with a history of fibrocystic disease of the pancreas may have congenital absence of the vas deferens, presumably resulting from a common genetic defect.

Urinary symptoms of an inflammatory or obstructive nature may be clues to a fertility-related problem. Patients with urethral stricture are more likely to notice their poor urinary stream than the retarded flux of their semen with its concomitant poor disposition.

By the same token, inflammatory symptoms of micturition may be more rapidly and more easily noticed by patients than the slightly painful ejaculation. These symptoms may occur in genital tuberculosis or in chronic recurrent vesiculo-prostatitis. Spermatogenesis may be affected by the intake of various pharmacological agents such as cytostatic or antimitotic drugs used not only for their immunosuppressive properties but also for the treatment of various non-cancerous diseases.

It is the intense mitotic activity of the postpubertal germinal epithelium of the testes that is most highly prone to damage from these drugs. Leydig cell function and testosterone secretion usually remain unimpaired under cytostatic treatment.

On the other hand, some drugs are known to interfere with Leydig cell function. Spironolactone inhibits testosterone synthesis by reducing testicular cytochrome P450 and 17 alpha-hydroxylase activity. The main antiandrogenic action of spironolactone seems to be its capacity to inhibit the binding of DHT to cytosol in nuclear receptors (Menard et al. 1978).

Acute and chronic alcohol consumption also appears to lower plasma testosterone synthesis. Moreover, ethanol increases the metabolic clearance rate of testosterone concomitant with an increase in hepatic 5 alpha-reductase activity and increased conversion of androgens into estrogens. Thus, testicular dysfunction may occur in patients prior to alcoholic liver cirrhosis.

The insecticide DDT competes for binding sites on the androgen receptor (Wakeling and Visek, 1973) and may exert some estrogenic effects.

Two other insecticides typically used against fire ants, Kepone (decachloro-octahydro-1,3,4-2H-cyclobutan-(cd)-pentalen-2-one) and Mirex, up to 10% of which is converted to Kepone, cause not only neurological damage but also testicular damage.

The suppressive effect of dibromochloropropane (DBCP) on human spermatogenesis was incidentally discovered in 1977. Epidemiological studies have indicated that factory employees exposed to this nematocide during its production developed oligozoospermia or azoospermia. Follow-up studies over a period of 8 years suggest that the gonadotoxic effect of DBCP might be reversible: This reversibility has been shown to be inversely related to previous exposure time and to most likely to occur in the presence of normal plasma FSH concentration. A marked increase in FSH and LH levels above the upper limit of normal was observed in those azoospermic workers in whom sperm concentration did not return to normal values. testosterone levels of all patients were normal at all times. Paternal exposure to DBCP was not associated with an increased risk for fetal malformations nor for spontaneous abortion (Potashnik & Yanai-Inber, 1987).

Also some tranquilizers, hypnotics, stimulants, phenacetin, salicylic acid derivatives, hormones, salazosulphapyridine, and nitrofurane as well as exposure to irradiation are known to interfere with fertility. It should also be remembered that various drugs increase plasma levels of prolactin, which may interfere with sexual potency and possibly fertility. Thus, a careful and extensive history of drugs and exposure to exogenous chemicals and/or irradiation may prove of importance in establishing the etiology of a fertility problem.

EXAMINATION OF THE INFERTILE MALE

The examining room should be warm so that the scrotal dartos reflex will be relaxed, facilitating the examination of the genitalia. It is, therefore, helpful to place a warm lamp near the scrotum during the examination.

The examination of the infertile man, in addition to a full physical examination, must include a meticulous investigation of the genital organs. Urogenital examination includes inspection of the penis and the location of the urethral opening. Any abnormalities concerning the prepuce should be noted. Palpation of the scrotal content provides information about localization, consistency, and possible tenderness of the testes. In order to measure the size of the testes, the scrotal skin is stretched over the testicle, and the contour of the testicle is defined by palpation and separated from the epididymal head. The size of the testicle is then compared to the corresponding ovoid on an orchidometer. Testicular size is an important clinical parameter for male infertility assessment.

Since 90–95% of the volume of a normal testis is made up of tubular tissue, the total testicular volume yields a good estimate of the amount of germinal epithelium. Men with small and firm testes (volume > 6 ml) may have Klinefelter's syndrome, a frequently overlooked chromosomal disorder. Testicular size of 15 ml or more is considered normal. Testicular size of less than 15 ml usually coincides with an abnormal spermiogram. Lack of usual firmness may indicate a loss of seminiferous epithelium (e.g. Sertoli cell only syndrome, Klinefelter's syndrome). The epididymis and vas deferens are carefully palpated in search of cystic formations, tenderness, or thickening which could confirm past, present, or chronic inflammatory disease resulting in infertility. The presence of scrotal swelling due to hernia or hydrocele is noted. With the patient standing upright, occurrence of varicocele or of spermatic venous reflux during the Valsalva maneuver is investigated.

Then the groin is examined for lymphadenopathy, surgical or other scars. Finally, prostate and seminal vesicles are examined. The prostate gland is easily palpated by rectal digital examination unless the patient is markedly obese. The knee-chest position is helpful in examining the obese patient. The prostate should be symmetrical, of firm consistency, normal in size, and not tender to palpation. Massage of the prostate is generally an uncomfortable procedure even to the normal male, and pain elicited by pressure to the prostate does not necessarily indicate that the gland is diseased. A prostate gland that is enlarged and boggy in consistency is often congested, infected, or both. Gentle massage of such a prostate may produce secretion which may reveal pus cells on microscopic examination.

The seminal vesicles cannot normally be palpated unless they are congested or diseased. The rust-colored semen occasionally noticed by patients is most often due to congestive seminal vesiculitis. Prostatic fluid and urine voided after prostatic massage should be examined and a bacteriological culture performed.

ENDOCRINE EVALUATION

An elevated prolactin level may be a symptom of hypothalamic inability to secrete the prolactin-inhibiting factor (PIF) or may be an early sign of pituitary adenoma.

The testosterone level should be determined in patients with history or signs of deficient development of the secondary sex characteristics and in men with sexual impotency. Sometimes the only sign of androgen deficiency may be deficient sperm motility or abnormal sperm output as a consequence of impaired epididymal sperm maturation. To determine the functional quality of the Leydig cells, the hCG stimulation test should be performed. The testosterone response to a single injection of 5,000 IU or an adjusted dose of 5,000 IU/1.7 m² as recommended by Tapanainen et al. (1983) for peripubertal boys is measured.   In hypogonadal males, a definite but sometimes reduced testosterone rise was observed in all patients within 48-96 h (mean 72 hours) (Forest and Roulier, 1982; Okuyama et al. 1981; Smals et al. 1979). We therefore take a blood sample at 72 h following a single hCG injection, with a repeated examination at 96 h to cover individual variations. If an enzymatic defect in Leydig cell function is suspected, the simultaneous measurements of androstendione and 17-hydroxyprogesterone levels will help to diagnose defects in 17-alpha-ketoreductase and 17-20-desmolase enzymes (Forest et al. 1980).

Testosterone, produced after hCG injection, stimulates seminal vesicles, epididymis, and prostate, and increases the concentration of their respective excretory products in seminal fluid. An increase in plasma testosterone without an increase in the concentrations of the physiological markers in the ejaculate indicates a mechanical block, dysfunction, or agenesis of the respective secondary sex gland.

Thus, the concomitant measurement of plasma testosterone and seminal fluid volume with its physiological markers following hCG stimulation (hCG-seminal plasma test) may help to precisely localize the lesion and aid in the diagnosis (Figs. 10-1, 10-2).

FSH determination is indicated in patients with a sperm concentration of less than 5 million per ml. Elevated levels indicate germinal cell insufficiency. In azoospermic men, high FSH levels indicate primary germinal cell failure, Sertoli cell only syndrome, or genetic conditions such as Klinefelter's syndrome. If elevated FSH levels are accompanied by elevated LH levels and subnormal testosterone, this indicates primary testicular failure, or 'andropause' (Lunenfeld et al. 1982). Elevated levels of LH in the presence of relative low values of testosterone are a sign of Leydig cell insufficiency. Administration of GnRH, a decapeptide that has been shown to stimulate the pituitary to synthesize and secrete both FSH and LH, may help to detect gonadotropic deficiency due to either pituitary insufficiency or secondary to long-standing hypothalamic insufficiency. Since inhibin secreted by the Sertoli cells inhibits GnRH-stimulated pituitary secretion of FSH, exaggerated FSH titers after GnRH stimulation indicate lack of inhibin. This in turn reflects an insufficiency of Sertoli cells and may also help to discover the patients with isolated primary germinal cell failure.

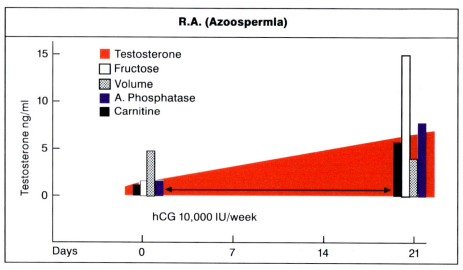

Fig. 10–1. The hCG-seminal plasma test: The effect of prolonged hCG stimulation on plasma testosterone, seminal fructose, acid phosphatase and carnitine concentration and seminal volume.

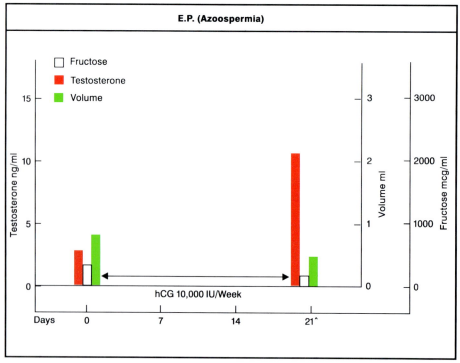

Fig. 10–2. The hCG-seminalplasma test: The effect of prolonged hCG stimulation on plasma testosterone and on seminal fluid volume and fructose concentration. Note lack of increase of fructose concentration.

We administer 100 µg of GnRH intramuscularly and measure FSH and LH levels twice prior to and at 15, 30, 90 and 120 minutes following injection. The results of the GnRH test are classified as follows:

Type 0:   Neither FSH nor LH levels increase (posthypohysectomy or primary pituitary failure). Such patients are suitable for gonadotropin therapy.

Type I: Base level of less than 1.5 mIU FSH with increase to less than twice the initial value and/or maximum FSH levels do not exceed 3 mIU/ml (relative pituitary insufficiency: usually secondary to long-standing hypothalamic insufficiency). hMG/hCG administration or pulsatile administration of GnRH is usually the treatment of choice for patients in this category.

Type II: FSH increases to less than three times the initial levels and maximum levels do not exceed 9 mIU/ml. This physiologic (normal) response is usually found in azoospermic patients with an occlusion of sperm-conveying structures. Such a response justifies a testicular biopsy to verify the diagnosis.

Type III: FSH increases more than three times the basal level and/or a maximum level exceeding 9 mIU/ml. This type of GnRH response is regarded as exaggerated and indicates Sertoli cell insufficiency or isolated masked germinal cell failure. No therapy is available in these cases (Fig. 10–3).

Each laboratory must establish its own normal values to make this test a useful tool for diagnosis.

In severe oligozoospermic males, determination of FSH should be performed. Increased levels may indicate a faulty pattern of GnRH release (Slow-pulsing Oligospermia – Wagner et al. 1985). This syndrome may be treated with pulsatile GnRH therapy (see Chapter 13).

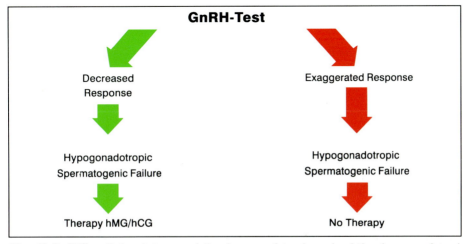

Fig. 10–3. Differentiation between relative hypogonadotropic and relative hypergonadotropic spermatogenic failure using GnRH.

11. SEMEN ANALYSIS

The most important single test in the evaluation of male infertility is the semen analysis. If performed skillfully and interpreted properly, it will provide a wide spectrum of information reflecting the spermatogenetic and steroidogenetic function of the testes and the functional state of the secondary sex glands (Glezerman & Bartoov, 1992).

COLLECTION OF THE EJACULATE

The patient should receive written guidelines giving exact instructions concerning sexual abstinence, collection, and transport of the sample. The only acceptable method for collection of the ejaculate is masturbation. Only this method permits complete collection of the specimen in a suitable container and best avoids contamination. The withdrawal technique is not very reliable, since some of the semen may be lost during withdrawal and vaginal secretions may contaminate the specimen. The use of commercially available condoms should be discouraged since these are coated with spermicidal substances. The specimen bottle, a wide-mouth container, should be supplied by the laboratory. It is advisable to use containers pretested by chemical and biologic studies as to their effects on seminal parameters. The screw top should not have any rubber lining, since contact with rubber may cause the death of sperm cells. The jar must be completely dry, since any water will quickly kill the spermatozoa (Jequier, 1986).

Sexual Abstinence Before Collection of the Ejaculate

The period of abstinence preceding collection of the semen specimen has a remarkable influence on spermatozoal concentration and a lesser effect on motility and morphology. There is a correlation between sperm concentration and the number of days of abstinence (Table 11–1). Schwartz et al. (1979) have found that each day of

TABLE 11-1. Relationship between Sexual Abstinence and Spermatozoal Concentration. Note that there is no further Increase of Spermatozoal Concentration after the 11th Day of Abstinence (Schirren, 1972)

Days of Abstinence	Mean Spermatozoal Concentration (x Mill./ml)	Days of Abstinence	Mean Spermatozoal Concentration (x Mill./ml)
1	13	8	105
2	31	9	96
3	53	10	227
4	82	11	166
5	86	12	146
6	96	13	152
7	87	14	161

abstinence increases the sperm count in healthy donors by 13 million cells per ml. For the sake of standardization, most laboratories specify a period of abstinence (usually 3–5 days). Sperm output observed in longitudinal studies may vary considerably even in fertile volunteers. Paulsen (1980) has followed the sperm output in one individual biweekly for 2 years. This healthy donor had no febrile illnesses during that period nor did he receive any medication. Sperm concentrations fluctuated between 5 million sperm cells per ml to 170 million/ml. Thus, examination of a single semen specimen is of very limited use in assessing the quantitative gametogenic function of the testes. Since both standardization and proper reflection of physiologic conditions are important in the evaluation of the infertile male, it is justified to perform 2–4 semen analyses prior to diagnosis and treatment. Motility seems to be much less dependent on abstinence and remains relatively stable, at least within a 5-day period. Sauer et al. (1988) used a method of automated videomicrography and measured five motility parameters in 10 fertile donors over a period of 120 hours. During this time period, no change in motility could be observed corresponding to changes in ejaculatory frequency. However, prolonged abstinence will result in the output of aging sperm cells from the epididymis with resultant decreased motility (Mortimer et al. 1982).

EXAMINATION OF THE EJACULATE

Usually the color of the ejaculate is whitish-gray to yellowish and tends more to yellowish the longer the abstinence period is. Discoloration of the semen may point to genital tract infections if the specimen appears white or yellow (leukocytes) or to bleeding from some point along the tract if the semen is reddish (erythrocytes). Finally, certain drugs such as antibiotics may lead to discoloration.

The odor of semen has been compared to chestnut flowers and results probably from the oxidation of spermine, which originates in the prostatic gland. The odor of semen may remind obstetricians of amniotic fluid.

Coagulation and Liquefication

Immediately after ejaculation, the liquid seminal fluid coagulates and subsequently liquefies within 5–40 minutes. The physiologic function of the process remains unclear (Lunenfeld and Glezerman, 1981). The coagulation process differs basically from blood coagulation as far as coagulation factors are concerned. The coagulative enzyme in man originates in the seminal vesicle while the liquefying enzyme, seminine, is produced by the prostate gland.

The progress of coagulation or liquefication may be disturbed. Azoospermia (i.e., complete absence of sperm cells in the semen sample) concomitant with complete lack of coagulation indicates agenesis of the seminal vesicle or occlusion of the ejaculatory ducts. If the seminal coagulum fails to liquefy, probably due to poor prostate lytic activity, the persistent coagulum may trap spermatozoa and restrict motility. Thus, observation of coagulation and liquefication is of considerable importance.

Following liquefication, the seminal fluid achieves a viscous state. Hyperviscosity may also impair sperm transport. Usually, viscosity is estimated by observing the ability of the fluid to adapt to the form of the slowly rotated semen container (Zaneveld and Polakoski, 1977) or by pouring it into another jar and observing its ability to fractionate (Amelar et al. 1977). A simple method involving centrifugation has been proposed (Boonsaeng, 1981). Based on the observation that only liquefying semen produces supernatant during centrifugation and that the amount of produced supernatant is directly related to the volume of liquefying coagulum, this method permits quantitative assessment of the seminal liquefication rate.

Volume and pH

Hypospermia and hyperspermia are terms describing semen samples with a volume of less than 1.5 ml or more than 5.5 ml, respectively. A man is considered aspermic if the sensation of orgasm is not accompanied by emission of semen.

The volume of the seminal fluid averages 2–5 ml. Prolonged sexual abstinence may result in a larger seminal volume. The prostatic and epididymal contribution to the seminal fluid does not usually exceed 1 ml. Thus, semen volume is mainly a function of the activity of the seminal vesicles. Inflammatory processes, mainly in this gland and to a lesser extent in the prostate, may lead to hyperspermia with resultant dilution of the cell content. Reduced seminal volume may be a sequel to chronic inflammatory processes in the prostate or seminal vesicles, may indicate androgen deficiency, may be the consequence of proximal occlusion of the ejaculatory ducts, or may reflect incomplete ejaculation or loss of parts of the specimen.

Determination of pH is easily performed using indicator paper. A pH exceeding 8.0 may suggest acute diseases of the seminal vesicles or may be due to delayed measurement. (Seminal plasma releases CO_2 continuously and, consequently, pH values increase as a function of time.) Low pH (< 7) may be a sign of occlusion of the ejaculatory ducts or of contamination of the semen specimen by urine or may indicate the presence of chronic inflammatory processes in the seminal vesicles.

Biochemical Evaluation of Semen

The seminal plasma is a confluent of secretions from epididymes, seminal vesicles, ampules, the prostate, and Cowper's and Littre's glands. A remarkable feature of the seminal plasma is the principal dependence of both its volume and chemical composition on the testicular hormone testosterone.

Visual and olfactory stimuli and erotic fantasies have been shown to increase testosterone production and consequently the activity of the secondary sex glands.

At the time of ejaculation, specific interactions between the secretions of the various contributing glands ensue. For instance, the seminal vesicles secrete a coagulable protein and the prostate provides the necessary liquefying enzyme. The epididymis secretes glycerylphosphorylcholine and phosphorylcholine and a prostatic acid phosphatase liberates free choline and inorganic phosphate. Spermine, derived from the prostate, forms crystals in a reaction with these phosphates.

Seminal plasma serves as a vehicle and diluent for spermatozoa and as a buffering medium protecting sperm cells from the hostile vaginal environment; it contains sources of energy and means to unlock energy-rich components of female genital secretions. These functions justify a deeper interest in seminal biochemistry on the part of those dealing with male infertility.

One of the most notable peculiarities of the seminal plasma is the high concentration of some uncommon organic substances and enzymes, such as fructose, citric acid, inositol, glycerylphosphorylcholine, acid phosphatase, 5-nucleotidase, and many others. For an excellent and exhaustive review, see Mann & Lutvak-Mann (1981).

Basic biochemical analysis of seminal plasma should include the assessment of markers for the functional state of the secondary sex glands and examination of substances that might be directly related to the possible fertilizing ability of the spermatozoa.

In this discussion we shall mention only a very selective and limited list of substances which may be assessed in a representative semen analysis. Specific tests, such as the histochemical enzyme examination, tests for acrosin activity and trypsin inhibitors, immunological tests, and others remain optional and are not part of routine semen analysis in most laboratories.

Epididymal Semen

Characteristic constituents of epididymal fluid are glycerylphosphorylcholine (GPC) and carnitine. Free choline in seminal plasma is a product of the breakdown of phosphorylcholine derived mainly from the seminal vesicle. In man, GPC, the typical epididymal product, is not easily metabolized in semen after ejaculation and may therefore serve as a marker for epididymal function. Jeyendran et al. (1989) have divided 52 men from an IVF program into one group of men whose sperm cells had fertilized ova and a second group in which no fertilization had been observed. GPC concentrations were significantly higher in the first group than in the second, suggesting that GPC may influence the fertilizing ability of sperm cells.

Yet, unlike those of most mammals, human seminal phosphatases are rather slow in metabolizing GPC, and its physiologic significance remains unclear.

Carnitine is a derivative of butyric acid and plays an important role in the transport of fatty acids through mitochondrial membranes and in regulating sperm fructolysis. Casillas (1973) has demonstrated that the carnitine content of bovine spermatozoa increases as they pass from the testes through the different parts of the epididymis. Carnitine may thus play a role in the maturation process of spermatozoa.

Wetterauer and Heite (1980) have measured carnitine obtained by an enzymatic-colorimetric method which specifically measures free carnitine. The authors concluded that 94% of free carnitine originates in the epididymis.

The role of carnitine as a specific epididymal marker is not sufficiently established and awaits further research. However, the suggested role of carnitine in the spermatozoal maturation process may justify its assessment in semen analysis.

Inhibin

This substance of testicular origin selectively suppresses the pituitary secretion of follicle stimulating hormone (FSH).

Several techniques have been employed to measure inhibin, most of them based on bioassay principles. Sheth et al. (1978) have proposed a radio-immuno-assay. Using this assay, Vaze et al. (1980) have measured levels of inhibin in seminal plasma of oligozoospermic and normozoospermic semen and in normal human accessory reproductive organs. Seminal concentrations showed positive correlation with sperm concentration. These authors were also able to demonstrate notable amounts of inhibin in seminal vesicles and prostate glands. The significance of this finding is still unclear.

In cases of azoospermia due to spermatogenetic failure, inhibin is absent from the seminal plasma (Scott and Burger, 1980). Assessment of inhibin may thus be a very valuable tool for prognosis of azoospermia. If, for instance, an azoospermic semen contains normal amounts of GPC but no inhibin, one may speculate that there is no obstruction but lack of spermatogenetic activity. The diagnosis of obstruction could be made if semen samples were found to be devoid of both GPC and inhibin.

Prostate Gland Fluid

The prostatic fluid is slightly acidic (pH 6.5) and particularly rich in enzymes. Acid phosphatase, beta-glucoronidase, lysozyme alpha-amylase, gamma-glutamyl-transferase, seminal proteinase (seminine), and other enzymes have been found. Other typical substances derived from the prostatic fluid are citric acid, calcium, zinc, and spermine, the latter being responsible for the typical odor of spermatic fluid. The ejaculatory process, initiated by contractions of the epididymis, is followed immediately by contractions of the prostate gland so that the first ejaculatory spurt, the so-called split, is composed of both epididymal and prostatic secretions.

Zinc

Compared to other body fluids and tissues, the concentration of zinc in seminal fluid is very high (15–30 mg% as compared to 75–115 mg% respectively).

Seminal plasma contains several zinc-binding ligands. It seems that some of them originate from the seminal vesicles (Arver, 1980). It has been reported that zinc taken up by spermatozoa during the contact of epididymal with prostatic secretions may be essential for an intrinsic sperm chromatin decondensation mechanism (Kvist, 1980). Unsaturated zinc-binding ligands from the seminal vesicle might reduce the bioavailability of zinc and thus decrease nuclear chromatin stability (Kvist and Eliasson, 1980). High levels of zinc ligands from the seminal vesicles or low levels of available zinc may thus influence spermatozoal nuclear chromatin stability. Zinc can be measured by atomic absorption spectroscopy. Since sperm cells are also rich in zinc, care should be taken that seminal plasma is devoid of sperm cells when tested for zinc.

Acid Phosphatase (AP)

Several acid phosphatases can be distinguished in the human testes (Guha & Vanha-Perttula, 1980). Most acid phosphatases, however, are secreted by the prostate gland; this substance is therefore a very reliable marker of prostatic function and has been used widely as a parameter for monitoring prostatic malignancies. One of the possible physiological functions of this enzyme is the breakdown of phosphorylcholine and the provision of free choline. No correlation between sperm count and motility, on the one hand, and AP, on the other hand, has been observed (Heite and Wetterauer, 1979). Among numerous methods of analysis, the method of choice is based on the enzymatic hydrolysis of the phosphate bond of p-nitrophenol (Polakoski and Zaneveld, 1977).

Seminal Vesicles

Immediately following the ejaculation of the epididymal prostatic spurt, the seminal vesicle contracts rhythmically and provides the remaining ejaculatory spurts. Some 70% of the seminal fluid originates in the seminal vesicles. The fluid is alkaline. The two best-known specific products of the seminal vesicle are fructose and prostaglandins. Although the seminal plasma contains a variety of sugars such as glucose, ribose, fucose, and others, fructose is the principal sugar providing a readily available exogenous energy source for sperm cells and presents a very specific marker for the functional state of the seminal vesicles. Levels above 1,200 mg/ml are considered normal. There does not seem to be a correlation between sperm count and motility and fructose levels (Videla et al. 1981; Glezerman et al. 1982). Among a variety of methods, fructose can be measured by gas chromatography (Ludwig et al. 1974), paper chromatography (Lewin and Beer, 1975), and colorimetric methods based on the resorcinol reaction (Mann, 1964). The latter method is probably the easiest and most widely applied.

Prostaglandins

The techniques available for measuring seminal prostaglandins are complicated and laborious. UV-absorption, densitometry, enzymatic analysis, gas chromatography with spectrometry, and radio-immuno-assay are some of the methods used. The determination of prostaglandins in seminal fluid is beyond the scope of the routine semen analysis. Yet the importance of these substances justifies a short discussion. Prostaglandins have been demonstrated in the epididymis and testes but the principal source of these long-chain fatty acids are the seminal vesicles. The human seminal plasma possesses the highest concentration of prostaglandins of all body fluids. Approximately 17 prostaglandins have been identified in seminal plasma. The most important of them being PGE(1) and PGE(2) and their 19–OH derivatives. Normal values are 30–200 mg/ml (PGE(1) + PGE(2)) and 90–260 mg/ml for the two derivatives respectively (Cooper and Kelly, 1975).

   The physiological role of prostaglandins in human semen is not yet clear. PGE stimulates adenylcyclase in most tissues. It is conceivable that seminal prostaglandins might raise the intraspermatozoal levels of cAMP, thus stimulating motility. Reduced prostaglandin levels in seminal fluid have been shown to be associated with male infertility (Collier et al. 1975).

Prolactin

Sheth et al. (1975) have demonstrated prolactin in the secretion of prostate and seminal vesicles. The level of prolactin in seminal plasma is 4–7 times higher than in blood serum. The physiological significance of this observation is not clear. Prolactin may influence sodium and potassium transport between spermatozoa and seminal plasma and thus influence sperm metabolism and motility. It has been stated that, in rats, prolactin, in addition to testosterone, stimulates prostatic function (Dattatreymurty et al. 1975). Analysis of prolactin is performed by radio-immuno-assay and is usually not part of a standard semen analysis.

MICROSCOPIC EXAMINATION OF THE EJACULATE

Before the microscopic examination is performed, it is absolutely necessary to have a well-mixed specimen. The easiest and quickest way is to use a vortex mixer for some 10 seconds at high speed. After liquefication, the sample should be checked microscopically for debris, bacteria, and epithelial and blood cells. Indication for bacteriological studies should be decided upon at this stage. The presence of immature cells should be noted and special attention should be paid to the presence of agglutination. Aggregation of sperm cells to cellular debris is not considered as agglutination. If more than 10% of sperm cells show head-head, tail-tail or head-tail agglutination, infection or immunological problems may be suspected and specific tests should be performed.

Sperm Count

The sperm concentration is usually determined either by using a hemocytometer (Burker chamber, Neubauer chamber), by using the Makler chamber (Makler, 1978), or by electronic counting methods, such as Coulter counters (Brotherton, 1979).

A semen sample in which, even after centrifugation, no sperm cells can be observed is termed azoospermic. Aspermia describes a condition in which no seminal fluid is discharged during orgasm. Oligozoospermia, normozoospermia, and polyzoospermia are terms defining semen samples containing less than the normal, normal, or higher than the normal concentrations of sperm cells respectively. There is no consensus, however, as to where the limits should be set (Table 11–2). Looking at the range of sperm counts in fertile men, i.e., men whose wives were pregnant at the time of semen analysis, men who have fathered at least two children and are applying for vasectomy, and fertile sperm donors, one finds sperm concentrations as low as 0.5

TABLE 11–2. Proposed normal Values for Sperm Concentration

Authors (Year)	Sperm Cells/ml (x Mill.)
Macomber and Sanders (1929)	60
MacLeod (1965)	20
Van Zyl (1972)	10
Santamauro et al. (1972)	10
Schirren (1972)	40
Schill (1975)	40
Ludvik (1976)	40
Freund and Petersen (1976)	40
Eliasson (1977)	20
Amelar et al. (1977)	40
Zaneveld and Polakoski (1977)	50
Zuckerman et al. (1977)	20
Brotherton (1979)	60
Homonnai et al. (1980)	10
Lunenfeld and Glezerman (1981)	30
Pryor (1981)	40

TABLE 11-3. Definitions of High Density Semen

Authors (Year)	Term	Sperm Density/ml (x 10^6)
Joel (1966)	Hyperspermia	120
Eliasson et al. (1970)	Polyspermia	250
Singer et al. (1979)	Polyspermia	200
Barnea et al. (1980)	Polyspermia	600 (mill/total vol)
Glezerman et al. (1982)	Polyspermia	250

million/ml (Homonnai et al. 1980). Bahamondes et al. (1979) reported the lowest concentration to be 2 million/ml, and Abylholm (1981) observed the same figure in his series.

Polyzoospermia is also only a poorly defined condition. Literature on polyzoospermia is scarce and the few studies dealing with it show a lack of standard criteria for diagnosis, different terms being used to describe semen samples with a sperm concentration considered to be higher than normal (Table 11-3). Patients with sperm concentrations above 250 million/ml seem to have impaired fertility.

Contemporary data reveal a peculiar downward shift in the average spermatozoal density in fertile men (Table 11-4). No study after 1974 showed an average sperm density above 100 million/ml in normal fertile men.

TABLE 11-4. Mean Spermatozoal Concentration in Men of Proved Fertility

Authors (Year)	Mean Sperm Count/ml (x 10^6)	No. of Men
Farris (1949)	145	49
Falk and Kaufman (1950)	101	100
MacLeod and Gold (1951)	107	1000
Sobrero and Rehan (1975)	81	100
Zuckerman et al. (1977)	63	4122
David et al. (1979)	98	190
Bahamondes et al. (1979)	68	186
Homonnai et al. (1980)	84	627
Abylholm (1981)	89	51
Jouannet et al. (1981)	95	324

Spermatozoal Motility

For the critical process of fertilization in the oviduct, few sperm cells are required; however, they must be motile. Therefore, one of the most important parameters in a semen sample is spermatozoal motility.

When evaluating motility, three parameters must be assessed: the percentage of motile cells, the type of motility, and longevity, i.e., the maintenance of spermatozoal motility as a function of time. Table 11-5 gives the mean percentage of motile sperm

TABLE 11–5. Mean Percentage of Motile Sperm Cells in Semen Samples of Men with Proved Fertility (Glezerman & Bartoov, 1986)

Authors (Year)	Mean % of Motile Cells	No. of Men
Falk and Kaufman (1950)	61	100
MacLeod and Gold (1951)	58	1000
Rehan et al. (1975)	65	1300
Bahamondes et al. (1979)	66	185
Homonnai et al. (1980)	49	627
Jouannet et al. (1981)	72	324

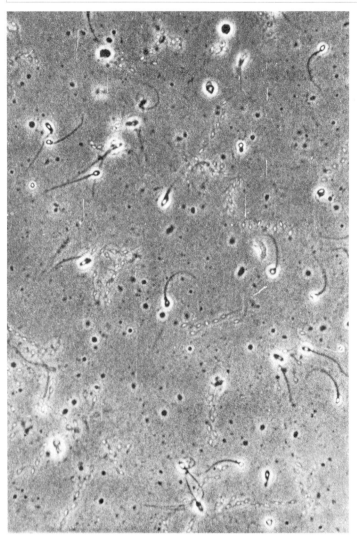

Fig. 11–1. Evaluation of sperm motility by multiple-exposure photography. For explanation see text.

cells in semen samples from men who had recently fathered a child, from men with at least two children who had applied for vasectomy, and from fertile donors. The average percentage of motility in these studies ranged from 49% to 72%. Based on these data, a semen sample containing more than 50% progressively moving sperm cells should be considered normal as far as motility is concerned.

Asthenospermia is a term which describes semen samples in which the percentage of motile cells is initially below 50%. Motility is generally evaluated by direct microscopic observation of the semen and is expressed in percentages. The type of movement (progressive or non-progressive) is assessed and the duration of motility is evaluated by repeated observation within a period of at least 3 hours. A motility loss of 10% – 20% within 3 hours is considered to be within the normal range.

The simplest and most widely used technique for the estimation of sperm motility is direct examination immediately following liquefication. This slide method has several drawbacks. It is subjective and no documentation can be kept. Percentage motility is usually overestimated, since spermatozoa that move in and out of the microscopic field may be counted several times, while the number of non-motile cells remains constant. Furthermore, the coverslip pressed on the drop is never absolutely parallel with the lower slide. A relationship between thickness of the examined drop and sperm motility has been demonstrated by Makler (1978b) and has been attributed to friction between sperm cells and the surface of the slide. The examination of different microscopic fields may therefore give markedly varying results and large errors in motility evaluation may occur.

Makler (1978a; et al. 1980) have reported on a method for a more objective determination of sperm motility. A special counting chamber of 10 µm depth was designed that provides standard conditions under which samples can be examined. Due to the special design of the chamber, vertical movement of cells and surface friction is eliminated while all cells are seen on one focal plane. Motility is measured by a multiple-exposure photographic technique (MEP) using a still camera and a stroboscope (Fig. 11–1). This system is also available in a computerized version for semi-automatic tracing. Other computerized systems have also entered the market (Hamilton-Thorn, Cellsoft).

Sperm Viability

When evaluating sperm motility, the percentage of moving sperm cells is determined and the characteristics of motion described. Non-moving sperm cells may be either dead or just 'dormant'. This distinction is essential if one plans to use in vitro vitalizing methods for subsequent artificial insemination. Assessment of sperm viability is based on supravital staining techniques. Several stains have been proposed, the most common of them being derivatives of fluorescein (eosin or erythrocin). Eosin in aqueous solution cannot penetrate living cells, and stained cells are therefore identified as being dead. Background stains, such as nigrosin, are often used in addition to permit easier identification of unstained (live) spermatozoa.

Equal parts of the staining solution (eosin solution in 0.15 molar phosphate buffer at pH 7.4) and semen (0.1 ml of each) are mixed thoroughly and, after 1–2 minutes, a drop of the mixture is transferred to a glass slide and allowed to air-dry. Examination is performed by means of a negative-phase contrast microscope. Viable sperm cells are bluish and dead cells appear bright yellow.

The percentage of stained cells (i.e., dead cells) is expressed as the percentage of eosin-positive cells.

Supravital staining may be useful also to identify cellular elements in semen. Precursors of spermatozoa are often mistaken for pus cells by technicians with little experience. Unnecessary antibiotic therapy is sometimes based on these erroneous test results.

Sperm Morphology

Mammalian spermatozoa possess a unique topography which clearly defines the various organelles responsible for the different functions the sperm cell must fulfill before and during fertilization. Generally, it is possible to assess the degree of maturation and integrity of sperm cells from surface microscopy using light and scanning electron microscopes. The unique, easily observable morphological features of the sperm cell and the ease of semen availability made the sperm morphogram one of the most powerful tools to infer the spermatogenic ability of the testes.

As many as 60 different morphologic forms of human spermatozoa have been reported (Brooks and Keel, 1979). In order to produce a workable morphogram, most laboratories dealing with routine semen analysis have adopted a simple classification system in which the sperm cell population is divided basically into normal and abnormal forms. The malformed spermatozoa are subdivided in up to 10 categories which can easily be defined with a certain degree of precision (duplicate head, tapering, large and small head, multitail, coiled tail defect, and proximal cytoplasmic droplet, etc.). The remainder of the malformed cells are usually 'dumped' (classified) in the 'amorphous' category (Zaneveld and Polakoski, 1977; Van Zyl, 1980; Eliasson, 1981).

The percentage of normal spermatozoa obtained from the population of fertile men in different laboratories ranges from 40% to 60%. This variance is probably due to varying staining techniques, the subjectiveness of observation, and the definitions of the malformations accepted by each semen analysis laboratory. Assessment of sperm morphology requires staining with fast-staining techniques, such as eosin-nigrosin (Blom, 1950), crystal violet (Brooks and Keel, 1979), or commercially available pre-stained slides (Calamera and Vilar, 1979). The Papanicolaou and Giemsa staining techniques for air-dried seminal fluid smear preparations are somewhat time-consuming and can be better used for differentiating between immature sperm cells, white or red blood cells, bacteria, epithelial cells, etc. We prefer the nigrosin-eosin technique since it is uncomplicated, it discriminates between the different regions of the sperm cell without causing shrinkage of the sperm head, and it provides information on sperm viability. The spermatozoa are observed under oil immersion at x 1,000 and the whole cell including head, midpiece, and tail is evaluated. Only when no malformation at all can be detected in the cell it is defined as normal.

It has to be borne in mind, however, that different staining techniques may produce a variation in results. Morphological data should be compared only when the staining technique is known and remains a constant. Furthermore, results obtained by light microscopy should not be compared to results obtained by electron microscopy (Glezerman, Bartoov, 1992). Using the latter method, the percentage of cells defined as normal are clearly the minority in any given semen sample (Table 11-6).

TABLE 11-6. Variations in Results of Sperm Morphology as related to Method applied

Method	Normal Forms
Bryan/Leishman	77.9 ± 9.7 (%)
Papanicolaou	49.8 ± 18 (%)
Eosin nigrosin	58 ± 15 (%)
SEM	30 ± 21 (%)
TEM	14 ± 8 (%)

A quantitative morphological method for evaluating the potential of the human testes to produce presumably fertile semen has been proposed (Bartoov et al. 1982). Instead of taking each morphological characteristic separately, a score is computed. This is a weighed sum of the original malformation measurements and is used to differentiate between a group of fertile men and a group of infertile men. The computation is based on the statistical discriminant analysis method (Nie et al. 1975).

Additional Tests

At least two additional tests should be mentioned here that may be used in selected cases to assess the biological behavior of sperm cells. The first is the Hamster egg assay and the other is the In vitro mucus sperm penetration test (see Chapter 8). Both tests may identify sperm pathology in semen samples that has remained undetected on routine examination. Insler et al. (1979) reported that 11.8% of men who had pathological mucus sperm penetration tests did not present any pathology in their routine semen analyses.

12. ALGORITHMIC APPROACH TO THE DIAGNOSIS OF MALE INFERTILITY

Methods for the precise localization of the lesions responsible for infertility have provided an impetus for transforming the treatment of male infertility from a largely empirical approach to a more logical one. On the basics of algorithmic schemes, infertile men can be classified into diagnostic groups depending on the etiology and on the location of the disturbance (Lunenfeld & Glezerman, 1977). This helps to designate the appropriate management for different diagnostic groups.

The experience of the physician will enable him to use short cuts, to focus attention to what is important and to add relevant extensions to the proposed scheme.

Results of at least two spermiograms should be available at the patient's first visit. Table 12-1 specifies the basic requirements of a semen examination and gives rough baselines for normal values.

An abundance of leukocytes or positive culture findings, i.e. pyobacteriosemia, mycoplasma, or chlamydia infections will point to urogenital inflammatory disease and further evaluation will be necessary (Fig. 12-1).

Table 12-2 lists guidelines for the diagnosis of secondary sex gland infections.

The patient's history may reveal environmental factors such as stress (Urry, 1977), toxic influences, or iatrogenic intervention, which may have led to what we have termed environmental oligo-terato-asthenospermia (OTA Syndrome) (Lunenfeld and Glezerman, 1977).

Detection of varicocele, hernia, or hydrocele (Fig. 12-2) will determine the therapeutic approach and the patient may be referred to surgery following the very first visit.

Biochemical evaluation of the seminal fluid and the use of specific markers may be helpful in locating a dysfunction along the genital tract (Table 12-3). Decreased values of either of these markers will require the hCG-seminal plasma test (see Chapter 10). The patient receives 5,000 IU human chorionic gonadotropin (hCG) twice weekly for 3 weeks. Testosterone levels are measured. The functional capacity of the androgen-dependent secondary sex glands is evaluated by measuring their secretory products. Persistent low levels of biochemical parameters may point to a secretory defect or, if co-existent with azoospermia, to a mechanical block at the corresponding topographic level. Normal increases of previously low levels of secretory products following the hCG medication will point to a relative androgen deficiency, which may be treated with hCG or mesterolone (Fig. 12-3).

AZOOSPERMIA

There are three distinct conditions characterized by semen void of sperm cells: (a) spermatogenic failure; (b) obstruction at any level of the genital tract; (c) ejaculative failure leading to relative retrograde ejaculation (Keiserman et al. 1974). The easily performed postcoital urine examination will exclude the latter variety.

On rare occasions, spermatogenic failure (azoospermia) coincides with the absence of scrotal testes. After having excluded a history of castration with subsequent androgen medication, the hCG-test will allow the detection of ectopic

TABLE 12-1. Guidelines for normal Values at Semen Analysis
(from Glezerman & Bartoov, 1992)

Observation

Volume	2–5 ml
pH	7.2–7.8
Color	Gray-white-yellow
Odor	Chestnut-like
Liquefication	Within 45 minutes

Sperm Cells

Sperm count	20–250 millions/ml
Sperm motility	> 50 % after liquefication
	> 40 % 3 hours later
Sperm morphology	
(light microscopy)	> 50 % normal forms
Eosin-positive cells	≦ 10 % stained cells

Biochemistry

Fructose	> 1200 µg/ml
Acid phosphatase	100–300 µg/ml
Citric acid	> 3 mg/ml
Inositol	> 1 mg/ml
Zinc	> 75 µg/ml
Magnesium	> 70 µg/ml
Prostaglandins	
(PGE 1 and PGE 2)	30–200 µg/ml
Carnitine	> 250 µg/ml
Glyceryl-phosphorylcholine	> 650 µg/ml

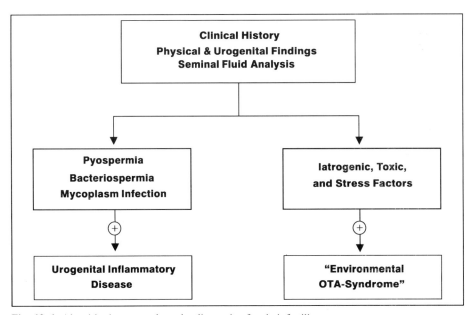

Fig. 12-1. Algorithmic approach to the diagnosis of male infertility.

TABLE 12–2. Criteria for Accessory Gland Infection

High pH	(7.8 – 8.1)
Low zinc	(8 – 14 mg/dl)
High PMN count	(> 3 / 5 HPF)

testes. If no testosterone rise occurs in a eunuchoid patient following hCG injections, one may conclude that no testicular tissue is present. However, these patients will usually not be able to produce any ejaculate.

The presence of scrotal testes in azoospermic patients requires a differential diagnosis between obstruction and testicular failure. To a certain extent, one may rely on the presence of seminal markers for the sexual glands in order to exclude obstruction. Vasography may be indicated in some cases while other cases may require testicular biopsy in order to prove intact testicular spermatogenesis, and by inference, obstruction of sperm-conveying structures.

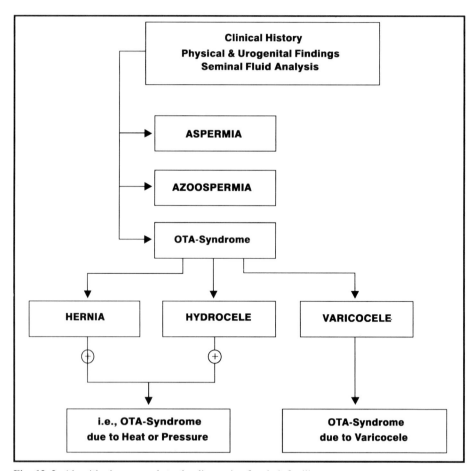

Fig. 12–2. Algorithmic approach to the diagnosis of male infertility.

TABLE 12-3. Localisation of Disturbances along the Male Genital Tract using Biochemical Markers of the Seminal Plasma

Carnitine GPC	Fructose	A. Phosphatase Inositol Sorbitol, Zn	Topography of Anatomic-Functional Impairment
+	+	–	Prostate
+	–	+	Seminal vesicles
–	+	+	Epididymis

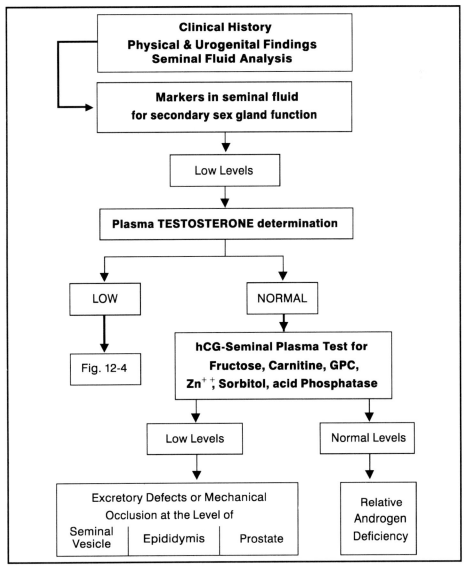

Fig. 12-3. Algorithmic approach to the diagnosis of male infertility.

In most cases, the determination of FSH levels will replace testicular biopsy. Elevated levels point to primary testicular failure, i.e. testicular atrophy, and chromosomal analysis may show a genetic syndrome, e.g. Klinefelter's Syndrome (Fig. 12–4). Negative genetic findings concomitant with elevated FSH levels point to conditions such as Sertoli-cell-only syndrome, focal tubular atrophy or spermatogenic arrest. In these cases, no therapy being available, testicular biopsy would be of academic interest only. If FSH levels have been found to be normal or decreased, one should perform a GnRH test. In azoospermic men, an exaggerated FSH rise is of the same diagnostic value as primary elevated FSH levels. If, on the other hand, FSH levels remain low or normal after GnRH administration, one may assume relative FSH deficiency, which may be treated by exogenous gonadotropins. Therapy has been reported to be successful in about 50% of these cases. This diagnostic approach is basically identical in patients whose testes have been found to be altered in size or consistency and who may present eunuchoid features. Low FSH levels in these patients point to secondary testicular insufficiency.

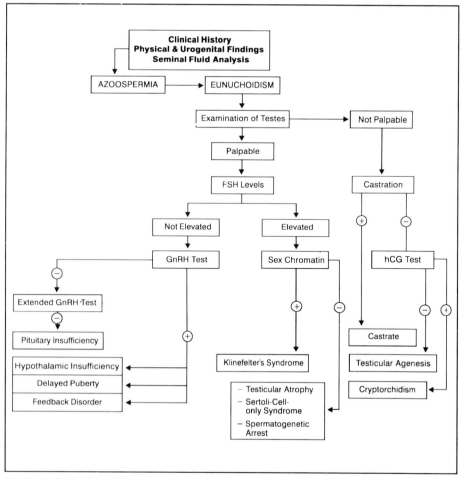

Fig. 12–4. Evaluation of the azoospermic male.

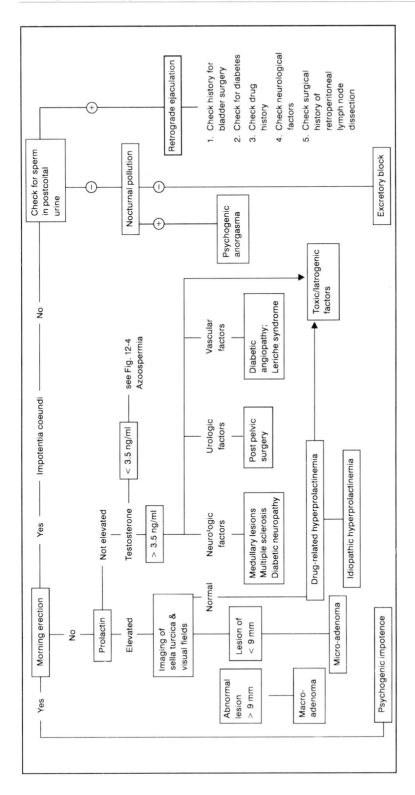

Fig. 12-5. Ejaculatory failure – In cases where erectory or ejaculatory insufficiency is accompanied by past or present signs of androgen deficiency, LH and testosterone determinations should be performed to assess the androgenic profile, and if androgen deficiency is confirmed, to localize its etiology. If LH is elevated in the presence of low or low-normal testosterone, primary Leydig cell insufficiency is most probably the cause. It should, however, be noted that elevated prolactin levels due to micro- or macro-adenoma may simulate such a condition. If LH and testosterone are low, pituitary insufficiency, hypothalamic-pituitary dysfunction, or the rare fertile enunch syndrome may be suspected. (From: Lunenfeld and Glezerman, 1982)

ASPERMIA

After endocrine causes of aspermia have been excluded, i.e. in eunuchoids, the diagnostic pathway for cases in which the ejaculatory deficiency occurs concomitantly with failure of erection differs from that for cases in which erection is intact. In the latter case (Fig. 12–5), one should primarily exclude retrograde ejaculation by examining postcoital urine samples (Glezerman et al. 1976b). If this syndrome has been excluded, the occurrence of nightly pollutions will point to psychogenic anorgasmia, while excretory block at the prostatic level may be assumed if nightly pollutions do not occur. Further evaluation, endocrinological as well as urological, is then necessary. Aspermia concomitant with erection failure may have a psychogenic background, i.e. psychogenic impotence. Usually, in these cases no morning erections are reported. On the other hand, if erections do not occur under any circumstances and psychogenic impotence has been ruled out, the patients should be evaluated for neurogenic factors, i.e. multiple sclerosis, diabetic neuropathy, urological factors such as the state following pelvic surgery, or vascular factors such as diabetic angiopathy. Finally, iatrogenic and toxic influences such as the use of certain anti-hypertensive drugs should be considered.

OTA-SYNDROME

We have labeled conditions in which a semen sample shows a decreased number of poorly motile and morphologically abnormal sperm cells Oligo-terato-asthenospermia (OTA-syndrome). Although all 3 of the above pathologies usually occur concomitantly, the degree of severity of each can differ significantly in various patients. In men with severe oligozoospermia, i.e. < 5 mill/ml, the GnRH test may reveal what we have termed masked hypergonadotropic hypogonadism. In some of these cases, pulsatile GnRH treatment may be successful (see "Therapeutic aspects").

In some patients, repeated seminal fluid analysis may show asthenospermia concomitant with a normal count and morphology, i.e. inherent motility deficiency (Fig. 12–6). If the eosin test indicates that most of the non-motile sperm cells are alive, in vitro treatment of spermatozoa by pharmaceutical (caffeine or kallikrein) or mechanical means (see "Therapeutic aspects") can be attempted. Subsequently, the treated sperm may be used for artificial insemination. In some cases in which in vitro vitalization has failed, hCG or androgen therapy may be beneficial. In these patients, the diagnosis of relative androgen deficiency may be established post hoc. Positive eosin test, i.e. more than 20% eosin-stained cells, will require a reevaluation of exogenous toxic influences.

In "dilution oligozoospermia" (oligozoospermia associated with a seminal volume of 3 ml or more) (Fig. 12–7), split sexual intercourse may enhance the chances of fertilization. If the relative concentration of morphologically abnormal forms is similar in both portions of the ejaculate, hMG/hCG therapy may occasionally prove beneficial. Those cases can be retrospectively classified as FSH deficient. Those who do not respond to hMG/hCG therapy are classified as idiopathic oligo-asthenospermic. Some of these may benefit from empirical treatment schemes (see Chapter 13).

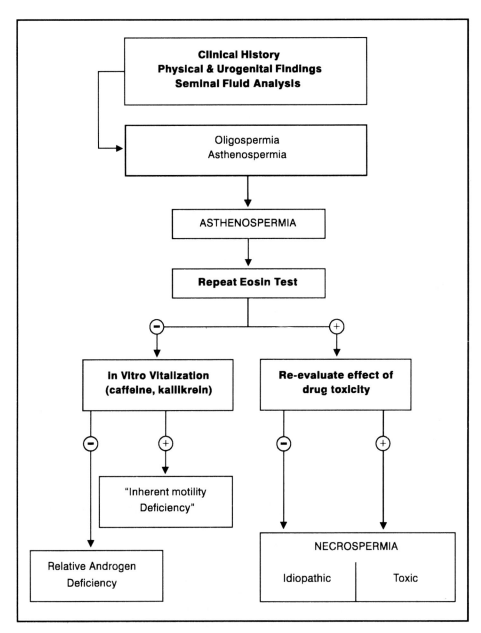

Fig. 12-6. Algorithmic approach to the diagnosis of male infertility.

Severe teratospermia, i.e. an ejaculate which contains more than 70% abnormal sperm cells, may be due to noxious influences or to chromosomal aberrations. A meticulous evaluation should be carried out.

It should be stressed that, in this chapter, no attempt has been made to cover the entire spectrum of the possible etiology of male infertility. The immunological aspect has not been elaborated and rarely encountered entities have not been mentioned.

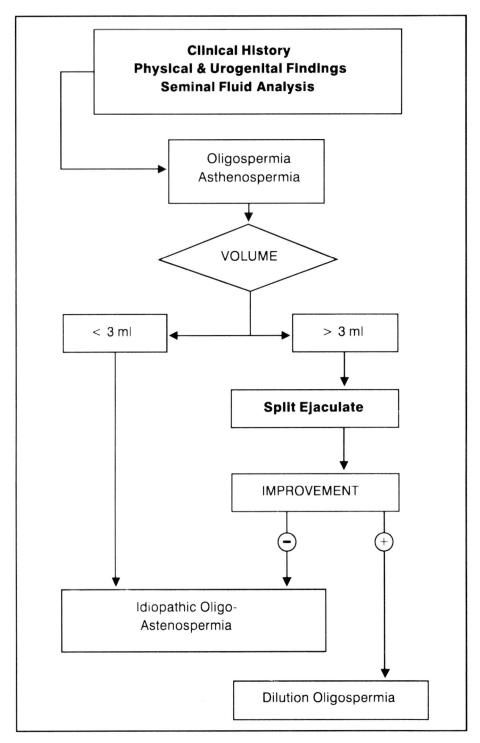

Fig. 12–7. Algorithmic approach to the diagnosis of male infertility.

13. THERAPEUTIC ASPECTS

Infertile men may suffer from erective, ejaculative, or spermatogenic dysfunction. As regards gonadotropin levels, these patients may be divided into 3 main groups: normogonadotropic, hypergonadotropic, and hypogonadotropic. Male infertility may be treated by drugs as well as by technical and surgical procedures. The algorithmic approach to the diagnosis of male infertility will enable the physician to define patients suitable for treatment and to choose the proper management in reasonable periods of time.

The hypogonadotropic patient may exhibit reproductive failure, coital failure, or both, depending on whether the condition interferes with the spermatogenic or the steroidogenic function of the gonads. In cases with a significant impedance of the latter function, poor development of the secondary sexual characteristics is usually evident.

Testicular failure may be primary or may be due to lack of stimulation by higher centers, i.e. secondary testicular failure due to hypothalamic or pituitary insufficiency. In the latter case, therapy aims at substituting the functions of the pituitary or hypothalamus. If testicular failure is not due to lack of stimulation but is primary, treatment should be symptomatic and restricted to substitution with androgens. Androgens will, in most cases, free the patient of the symptoms of androgen deficiency, induce and maintain development of secondary sexual characteristics, ensure a satisfactory sex life, and enable the patient to socialize normally.

Failure of spermatogenesis resulting from primary germinal failure or due to primary testicular dysfunction cannot be cured to date. If this condition is concomitant with hypoandrogenism, substitution therapy with androgens may be indicated. Patients over the age of 40 receiving chronic androgen therapy should be periodically examined in order to detect early signs of stimulation of a prostatic microcarcinoma.

Typical examples of hypergonadotropic hypogonadism are chromosomal aberrations such as Klinefelter's syndrome (Klinefelter et al. 1942), primary tubular failure such as Sertoli-cell-only syndrome (Del Castillo et al. 1947) and irreversible tubular damage, e.g. following mumps orchitis. Normogonadotropic azoospermic males who respond to GnRH administration with an exaggerated rise of FSH titers should also be included in this group.

GONADOTROPHIN-RELEASING HORMONE (GnRH)

Therapy with GnRH should, logically, be the treatment of choice in hypothalamic failure. Early reports on treatment with GnRH were disappointing. The commercially available native synthetic GnRH possesses a very short biological half-life (4–9 min.), and repeated daily applications were required. Development of long-acting analogs with greater potency led to renewed attempts at treatment but the now well-recognized phenomenon of down-regulation defeated this treatment modality. The realization of the pulsatile nature of GnRH and gonadotropin secretion and the experience gained in the treatment of female infertility using pulsatile applications of GnRH (Chapter 4) has been adopted in the treatment of male infertility. Results reported to date are promising (Jacobson et al. 1979; Valk et al. 1980, Skarin et al. 1982; Aulitzki and Frick, 1985). Shargil (1987) compared twice-daily subcutaneous injections with continuous subcutaneous injections via an infusion pump in 30 men with hypogonadotropic hypogonadism. The pulsatile treatment was found to be superior in terms of endocrine responses, spermatogenesis, and the fertilizing capacity of the newly-produced sperm. Full spermatogenesis has been induced in hypogonadotropic males and conceptions have been reported (Crowley, 1988; Berezin & Lunenfeld, 1988). Wagner et al. (1985) have described a condition which they termed "Slow pulsing oligospermia". The salient features of this syndrome are severe oligozoospermia associated with elevated FSH levels and low frequency of LH pulses. Pulsatile GnRH treatment resulted in normalization of FSH levels and increase in sperm density.

HUMAN MENOPAUSAL AND CHORIONIC GONADOTROPHIN (hMG/hCG)

Hypogonadotrophic hypogonadism involving both the steroidogenic and the spermatogenic compartment of the testes is exhibited clinically as eunuchoidism. Isolated FSH deficiency in the presence of normal FSH levels has been reported occasionally. Isolated LH deficiency with normal FSH levels may be found in the fertile eunuch syndrome (Makler et al. 1977). Ideal treatment of hypogonadotropic hypogonadism aims at complete restoration of testicular function, i.e. normal spermatogenesis and steroidogenesis. Selection criteria for the treatment of such patients are shown in Table 13-1.

The usual treatment schedule consists of testicular priming by 1-2 weekly hCG injections (5,000 IU). The aim is to achieve maturation of Leydig cells that will produce sufficient amounts of testosterone. After 4-8 weeks' treatment with hCG, hMG is instituted while hCG treatment is maintained. Various treatment schedules have been proposed. Sherins et al. (1977) assessed the minimal requirements for FSH to induce spermatogenesis in men with extreme hypogonadotrophism. Nine males received 2,000 IU of hCG 3 times weekly for at least 1 year. Thereafter, increasing

TABLE 13-1. Treatment with Human Menopausal Gonadotrophins; compiled data from the literature (based on reviews by Rosemberg 1976; Glezerman et al. 1978 and Schill 1986)

Group	No. of Patients	* Complete Spermatogenesis ** Improvement to > 30 Mill./ml
Hypophysectomized males	26	* 26 (100 %)
Hypogonadotrophic hypogonadism	38	* 32 (82 %)
Non-eunuchoidal azoospermic males	132	* 63 (48 %)
Severe oligozoospermia (< 10 Mill./ml)	439	** 78 (18 %)
Moderate oligozoospermia (< 20 Mill./ml)	241	** 35 (14.5 %)

dosages hMG was co-administered with hCG. Treatment was monitored by measuring plasma gonadotropins, plasma testosterone, testicular size increasing and sperm output. The authors concluded that spermatogenesis may be induced in hypogonadotropic males using only 10-30% of the conventional FSH dosage.

We use daily applications of hMG, starting with 75 units FSH (= 1 ampoule) per injection. This treatment schedule is continued for at least 3 months. The dosage may then be increased if spermatogenesis has not been initiated. In some cases dosages of to 300 IU FSH may be required. After spermatogenesis has been induced, in some cases it may be maintained with hCG alone. In effect, in some patients hCG treatment may be sufficient for inducing and maintaining spermatogenesis despite undetectable FSH levels (Levalle et al. 1984). HCG treatment has also been used successfully in maintaining spermatogenesis after induction with pulsatile GnRH treatment (Morris et al. 1985).

hMG/hCG treatment has been highly successful in men following hypophysectomy and in men with hypogonadotrophic hypogonadism. In our own series, 28 of 38 azoospermic patients (74%) who exhibited low FSH and low testosterone levels responded with full spermatogenesis, and 22 of them sired 39 children.

Noneunuchoidal azoospermic men showed a much lower degree of responsiveness to this mode of treatment. In oligozoospermic patients, results are discouraging (Table 13-1).

It is possible that the poor results obtained with hMG/hCG therapy in oligozoospermic men are due, at least in part, to inaccurate selection of patients. A very careful selection may help to identify that small segment of the oligozoospermic group, that might benefit from gonadotropin therapy (Schill et al. 1982). In carefully selected patients with relative FSH deficiency, who may sometimes be diagnosed with the help of the GnRH test (see Fig. 12-4), hMG/hCG may be an effective treatment.

Results of treatment with hCG alone for oligozoospermic patients have been equivocal (Mehan & Chehval 1982; Margalioth et al. 1983).

In isolated asthenospermia, positive results of treatment with hCG have been observed (Pusch et al. 1986a).

CLOMIPHENE CITRATE

Clomiphene citrate (CC) is a synthetic analog of the non-steroidal estrogen chlorotrianisene (TACE). Its mode of action is described in Chapter 5. The high efficiency of CC in the treatment of anovulation has led to various attempts to employ CC in the treatment of male infertility.

At present, it is difficult to clearly define patients who will respond favorably to treatment with CC. A controlled double-blind study showed CC to be efficient in men with decreased base levels of FSH and stressed the use of low-dosage treatment for at least 3 months (Roennberg, 1980). Micic and Dotlic (1985) have performed a randomized trial with CC and placebo in 101 oligozoospermic males with low-normal FSH levels. Statistically significant improvement in sperm parameters occurred in the treated group. Pusch et al. (1986b) reported similar results in a comparable group of 30 patients. While treatment with CC had no apparent effect on motility and morphology, sperm density increased significantly following treatment with 25 mg CC/day for 4 months.

Schellen (1982) and Schill (1986) have compiled results from the literature. Out of 574 men who were treated with low-dose CC (25 - 50 mg/d), improvement in sperm count was observed in 289 (50%) but only 69 men (14%) reported pregnancies. The substantial differences in results between the various reports are probably due to patient selection, duration of treatment, dosage, and additional factors that may contribute to infertility. It seems, however, that careful selection of patients with emphasis on low-normal basic FSH levels, the use of low-dosage (25 50 mg/d), and prolonged treatment (at least 3–4 months) may have some merit in the treatment of the OTA syndrome.

TAMOXIFEN

Tamoxifen is structurally similar to clomiphene citrate. It contains only one isomer, in contrast to CC, which is a racemic mixture of equal parts of trans isomers and cis isomers. The mode of action is similar to that of CC (see Chapter 5). On the hypothalamic level, tamoxifen interferes with the negative feedback by estrogen and activates GnRH release. Some studies published have reported favorable results as far as increase of sperm count is concerned (Buvat et al. 1982; Krause et al. 1985; Lewis-Jones et al. 1987; Schieferstein et al. 1987; Schill and Landthaler, 1980). Pregnancy rates reported by these authors were in the 30–35% range. Concerning motility, results have been equivocal. Noteworthy is that, in the only double-blind cross-over study reported to date (Ainmelk et al. 1987), tamoxifen was not more effective than placebo.

ANDROGENS

It has been shown (Steinberger, 1977) that the intratesticular concentration of testosterone required for the maintenance of spermatogenesis is approximately 50 to 100 times higher than the concentration of this steroid in peripheral blood. The differential gradient is maintained by an intratesticular androgen-binding protein (ABP).

Theoretically, exogenous administration of testosterone for the treatment of male infertility should be considered a self-defeating proposition. In order to attain in peripheral blood testosterone concentrations similar to those observed in the testes of normal males, exceedingly high doses of the drug must be administered. In this situation, adequate amounts of androgen-binding protein would not be available and a great part of the hormone administered would remain in the form of free testosterone. This may exert toxic effects as well as causing damage to the tubular architecture. Moreover, testosterone may suppress GnRH and consequently gonado-tropin secretion. Atrophy of the germinal epithelium may result. Yet, some reports have claimed satisfactory clinical results with (oral) testosterone undecanoate (Franchi et al. 1978).

The so-called rebound therapy, aiming at reducing spermatogenesis to azoosper-mic levels with subsequent rebound effect, has been disappointing. In normal men participating in trials for male fertility control, rebound effects have not been observed (Patanelli, 1978). Nieschlag and Freischem (1982) have compiled data from the literature. In the partners of 1,470 men who participated in 5 representative trials using testosterone rebound therapy, the pregnancy rate was 17%. This rate is within the rate of spontaneous pregnancies reported by patients with OTA syndrome. We feel that the efficacy of treatment with parenteral or oral preparations of testosterone is presently equivocal at best. We do not employ testosterone in the treatment of male infertility and we restrict this treatment to patients in whom the spermatogenic testicular compartment can be neglected (hypergonadotropic hypogonadism, castrates, or patients with hormonal impotence who do not desire children).

MESTEROLONE

Mesterolone (Fig. 13–1) is an orally effective androgen derivative which is not aromatized to estrogen due to a methyl-group at carbon 3. Since central negative feedback is exerted most probably by estrogen, no depression of gonadotropic activity has been observed in patients treated with this drug at dosages of up to 100 mg daily.

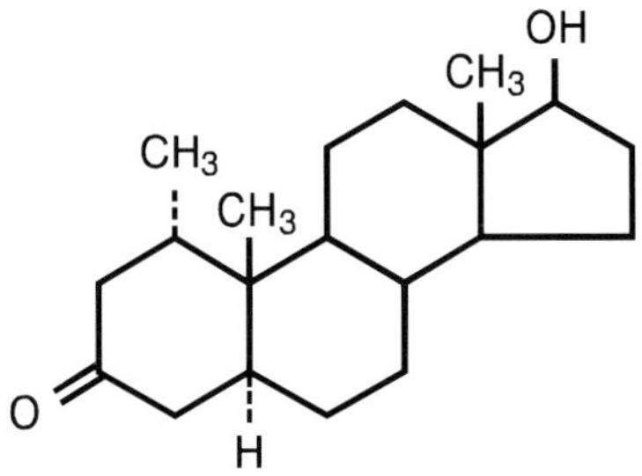

Fig. 13–1. Chemical structure of Mesterolone.

Yet Santen (1975) has shown that, while estrogens reduce the amplitude of LH pulses, both aromatizable and non-aromatizable androgens may reduce their frequency. While some authors (Schellen, 1970; Mauss, 1974; Glezerman et al. 1978) have reported that treatment with mesterolone is effective in idiopathic oligozoospermia, others (Somazzi et al. 1973) did not observe this effect. No distinct group of patients can be defined who may profit from this therapy, although, in some cases of relative androgen deficiency, mesterolone may be beneficial. Since this drug exerts little if any hepatotoxicity (Giarola, 1974), empirical use may be indicated, especially in cases of idiopathic asthenospermia.

TESTOSTERONE UNDECANOATE

Testosterone undecanoate (TU) is an oral testosterone preparation used for testosterone supplementation in hypogonadotropic males (Mies and Krempl, 1980; Maisey et al. 1981). The long-term safety of this drug has been established by Gooren (1986). Pusch (1989) reported on a double-blind study using 120 mg/d TU for 100 days in 60 men. While sperm motility remained unchanged following treatment, sperm morphology improved significantly.

ANTIBIOTICS

Acute or chronic infections of the secondary sex glands may result in morphological changes of the sperm cells, may impair prostatic and seminal vesicle function, and may even lead to occlusion of the excretory and ejaculatory ducts. The presence of pathogenic microorganisms can not always be demonstrated due to the bactericidal properties of seminal fluid. Baker et al. (1979) and Nikannen et al. (1979) have reported improvement of seminal parameters after antibiotic treatment even if no pathogens were demonstrated in seminal fluid. We usually rely on the criteria listed in Table 12-2 for the diagnosis of infection of the accessory glands. It has been shown that doxycycline (Oosterlinck et al. 1976) and trimethoprim-sulfamethoxazole (Gnarpe and Friberg, 1976) achieve high concentrations in the fluids of the seminal vesicle and the prostate gland. These drugs are therefore often used in the treatment of infections of the secondary sex glands.

OTHER APPROACHES TO MEDICAL TREATMENT OF MALE INFERTILITY

Various systemic therapies using thyroid hormones (Stewart and Montie, 1973), corticoids (Michelson et al. 1955; Hotchkiss, 1972), Vitamin E (Bartak, 1974), and arginine (Jungling and Bunge, 1976; da Rugna and Stahel, 1976) have been tried in the treatment of male infertility without apparent success.

Sperm-vitalizing Therapy

Various in vitro methods have been described that aim to improve the quality of sperm cells for subsequent insemination. Basically these methods add chemical compounds to semen or use mechanical means to attempt to separate quantitatively inferior cells from the superior portion.

Compounds

Kallikrein (Schill et al. 1974) or caffeine (Schoenfeld et al. 1975) have been employed in the treatment of asthenospermia. Kallikrein, a proteinase, releases kinins which enhance sperm metabolism. Some authors (Schill, 1975a) advocate the addition of blood serum as a source of kininogen.

Schill et al. (1974) observed enhancement of sperm motility after adding kallikrein to semen samples of asthenospermic males. Motility was increased in vivo by over 100% in 21 out of 57 patients after parenteral treatment with kallikrein for seven weeks (Schill, 1975b).

Caffeine inhibits cyclic nucleotide phosphodiesterase, thus preventing degradation of cyclic nucleotides which stimulate sperm metabolism. In vitro results using this approach have been rather positive. Haesungsharern and Chulavatnatal (1973) found that caffeine, theophylline, and aminophylline stimulate the motility of human spermatozoa in vitro. The percentage of motility increased and the mean motility rate was doubled. Johnsen et al. (1974) confirmed these findings. However, data reported by Doughtery et al. (1976) contradicted these reports and suggested that methylxanthins do not have beneficial effects on the majority of semen samples. Moreover, in some individual semen samples that responded favorably to caffeine and theophylline, sperm motility appeared to be jittering and not a normal type of motion.

Mechanical Methods

Glass Wool Columns

Paulson et al. (1979) have reported that passing a semen sample through glass wool columns may remove debris and immotile cells. The passage caused a loss of some 60% of cells but resulted in a sample with a high percentage of motile cells.

Albumin Columns

Albumin in concentrations between 7.5% and 17.5% has been used to separate high-quality sperm cells from immotile and morphologically abnormal cells (Dmowski et al. 1980). Various albumin concentrations have been used, and one- to three-layer columns have been employed in order to enhance the efficiency of separation and to reduce as much as possible the loss of cells. Typically between 40% and 80% of the cells will be lost during passage through albumin columns. The rate of loss may be reduced by using lower concentrations of albumin. Paz et al. (1986) used single-layer columns and Urry et al. (1983) increased the incubation period in order to reduce loss of sperm cells.

Other Filtration Columns

A variety of substances has been used to separate qualitatively inferior sperm cells from morphologically intact and motile spermatozoa. Kaneko et al. (1983) and Pardo et al. (1988) have used percoll. Quinlivan et al. (1982) have applied sephadex and Gellert-Mortimer et al. (1988) have proposed nycodenz gradients.

Centrifugation and Sperm Rise Techniques

Jeulin et al. (1982) have observed that centrifugation of sperm cells at 260 g did not have adverse effects. Centrifuging sperm cells and replacing the supernatant plasma with a nutrient such as Eagle's solution, Tyrode's solution, or HAM F-10 medium allowed motile and optimally configured cells to swim away from the pellet and concentrate in the nutrient solution, from where they can be retrieved. This method, like the methods using columns, is associated with a high loss of sperm cells and aims to replace quantity with quality.

CORRECTIVE SURGERY

Among men consulting an infertility clinic, some 3% exhibit azoospermia due to obstruction (Wagenknecht, 1982). Ductal obstruction or congenital anomalies of sperm-conveying structures have been treated by vaso-vasostomy, epididymo-vasostomy, etc. The most common indication for corrective surgery is reversal of vasectomy. As far as patency is concerned, results of microsurgery for this indication are excellent (Table 13-2). Epididymo-vasostomy has been less successful but is still indicated in selected cases of iatrogen or acquired obstruction (Table 13-3). As a last chance, alloplastic sperm reservoirs have been produced for subsequent aspiration of sperm cells and artificial insemination (Wagenknecht et al. 1980).

TABLE 13–2. Results of Vaso-Vasostomies

Authors (Year)	No. of Cases	Patency (%)	Pregnancies (%)
Derrick et al. (1973)	1630	30	19.5
Dorsey (1973)	129	88.3	18
Amelar and Dubin (1975a)	93	84	33
Schmidt (1975)	117	80	30
Lee (1976)	185	81	35
Wagenknecht (1982)	56	76	18

TABLE 13–3. Results of Epididymo-Vasostomy (modified after Schmidt et al. 1977)

Author	Cases	Patency	Pregnancies
Hagner	85	26	20
Bayle	178	130	89 of 56 couples
Joel	14	8	6
Fogh-Anderson & Hammen	30	14	6
Pomerol	43	18	4
Schoysman	72	38	10 (5-years follow-up)
Schoysman	184	79	31 (1-year follow-up)

(The references list for this Table can be obtained from the authors.)

VARICOCELE (VC)

Although varicocele has been known as a clinical condition for almost 2,000 years (Hotchkiss, 1970), it was only about 40 years ago that a patient was treated for his varicocele in order to restore (successfully) fertility (Tulloch, 1952). Today, it is estimated that some 20,000 males per year undergo correction of varicocele in an attempt to restore fertility (Turner, 1983).

Diagnosis of Varicocele

The clinical diagnosis of a VC is based on inspection and palpation. We have found the classification by Uehlig (1968) rather useful:

Stage I: No VC on inspection and palpation, but palpable filling of the pampiniform plexus during a valsalva maneuver.

Stage II: No VC on inspection, but detectable VC by palpation.

Stage III: VC clearly visible.

Other means for diagnosis of a VC are scrotal thermography, Doppler echography, venous scintigraphy, and retrograde venography.

Etiology of Varicocele

Nearly 98% of varicoceles are detected on the left side. This is due to the fact that, while the right spermatic vein enters the vena cava in an oblique fashion, the left spermatic vein enters the renal vein at a sharp angle. Continuous hydrostatic pressure due to man's upright position, congenital or acquired insufficiency or absence of venal valves, and the double 90° turn which venous blood from the spermatic vein has to take in order to reach the caval vein may all contribute to the formation of venal dilatation in the left spermatic vein and the formation of a varicocele. Furthermore, Sayfan et al. (1984) have described what they termed a nutcracker phenomenon: the superior mesenteric artery impinges on the renal vein and causes a rise in the intravascular resistance in this vessel. This renders the drainage of venous blood from the spermatic vein into the renal vein more difficult and may contribute to the dilatation of the pampiniform plexus.

Pathophysiology of Varicocele-Associated Infertility

The temperature within the scrotum is some 2.2 °C lower than the core body temperature. Any increase of temperature in the spermatogenetic environment caused by a large varicocele containing slow-moving venous blood may impair spermatogenesis. Yet it seems that no correlation exists between the size of varicocele and the prognosis following treatment of VC. Thus, the presence of a small varicocele may also be detrimental to intact spermatogenesis. The reasons for this finding may be manifold. Stasis of blood in the internal spermatic vein may lead to local hypoxia; reflux of toxic substances from the renal vein and the adrenal vein may interfere with spermatogenesis; and epididymal function may be impaired by the same mechanisms. Finally, these mechanisms may cause altered hormone production in the Leydig cells (Hudson, 1988). Cockett et al. (1984) observed a decrease in testicular size when the presence of varicocele was associated with impairment of seminal parameters. These authors have proposed treating a varicocele in an infertile man if more than 20% of the sperm cells are immature or have a tapered configuration and when there is a reduction in testicular size.

Treatment of Varicocele

While some investigators feel that treatment of varicocele in an infertile male does not enhance fertility, most studies have shown an amelioration in sperm parameters after treatment for VC and an increased pregnancy rate in the respective female partners (Table 13–4).

The treatment of a varicocele should be reserved for those patients who complain of local discomfort or in whom infertility is associated with impaired seminal parameters. There is no clear evidence that prophylactic treatment of varicocele is justified. Glezerman (1984) summarized surgical techniques currently in use for the treatment of varicocele. The most commonly used technique, introduced by Ivanissevich and Gregorini (1918), is based on suprainguinal (high) ligation of the spermatic vein. Non-surgical techniques have been introduced during the past decade and are based on selective catheterization of the left internal spermatic vein and the introduction of sclerosing substances or foreign bodies such as balloons, coils, springs, and gelfoam sponges into the vein (Glezerman and Jecht, 1984). The observation period after a varicocele operation should be restricted to 9 months, in which about 75% of the expected improvement takes place (Glezerman et al. 1976a).

TABLE 13-4. Pregnancy Rates after Treatment of Varicocele

Authors (Year)	No. of Men	Semen Analysis Improvement (%)	Pregnancy Rate (%)
Tulloch (1952)	30	66	30
Scott (1961)	93	78	29
Hanley & Harrison (1962)	78	68	28
Scott & Young (1962)	142	70	30
Charny & Baum (1968)	104	61	24
Brown et al. (1968)	185	60	43
MacLeod (1969)	108	74	40
Kaufman et al. (1974)	80	85	26
Brown (1976)	251	58	41
Dubin & Amelar (1977)	986	70	53
Lome & Ross (1977)	80	78	51
Homonnai et al. (1980)	238	50	40
Newton (1980)	149	55	34
Mattei et al. (1981)	140		38
Abdelmassih et al. (1982)	220	75	40
Soffer et al. (1983)	55		62
Cockett et al. (1984)	130		46
Glezerman (1984)	99	47	40
Menchini-Fabris (1985)	123	78	57
Total	3355	66.6	43.4

(The reference list for this table can be obtained from the authors.)

"SPLIT" INTERCOURSE

Approximately 30% of the ejaculate consists of prostatic gland secretions, spermatozoa, and epididymal fluids while the remaining 70% originates in the seminal vesicles. During the ejaculatory process, prostatic secretions and spermatozoa mixed with epididymal fluid are produced first. Subsequent emissions are composed mainly of secretions derived from the seminal vesicle. Consequently, the portion resulting from the first ejaculative contraction will contain the highest density of sperm cells (usually with a higher percentage of motile sperm cells than in the following spurts). This first split may then be used for insemination or the husband may be instructed to practice coital withdrawal after the deposition of the first split of the ejaculate. Results of this technique in oligozoospermic patients have been favorable (Amelar and Dubin, 1975).

14. THERAPEUTIC INSEMINATIONS

Therapeutic inseminations may be performed using either the husband's semen (AIH) or semen from a fertile donor (AID).

When medicinal, surgical, and other treatment schemes have failed, an attempt may be made to employ artificial insemination procedures.

TECHNIQUE OF ARTIFICIAL INSEMINATION

Artificial insemination may be accomplished by means of semen deposition in the vagina, around the cervix, into the cervix, or into the uterus. Special insemination instruments such as cervical caps are available.

Timing of Insemination

The life span of the human ovum is believed to average 6–24h, while motile human sperm cells have been observed in the cervical mucus for periods up to 205h following sexual intercourse. Thus 2 to 3 inseminations per cycle on alternative days will usually suffice to "cover" the periovulatory period and ensure that sufficient sperm cells are available at the fertilization site when the ovum arrives. If necessary and available, serial assays of LH and/or E2 and sonographic scans of the ovary may help in accurate determination of the ovulation day. With exact timing of ovulation, a single insemination per treatment cycle may be sufficient.

HOMOLOGOUS INSEMINATION

Indications

Mere substitution of the natural sperm-delivery mechanism by mechanical means (e.g., vaginal insemination) does not ameliorate the decreased fertilizing capacity of a given semen. Only if artificial insemination can provide additional protective, promotive, or corrective features will its use be superior to sexual intercourse for procreative purposes.

Male Factors

Hypospermia

Hypospermia is defined as a condition in which repeated semen analysis reveal a seminal volume of less than 1.5 ml. In cases of severe hypospermia, i.e., seminal volume below 1 ml, infertility may be due to the failure of the small amount of seminal fluid to make contact with the cervical os and its secretions. In these cases protective AIH may improve the fertilizing ability of the semen sample. One may either use commercially available cervical caps or perform intra-pericervical AIH.

Oligozoospermia

In cases of isolated oligozoospermia, a rational approach is to concentrate as many as possible of the available spermatozoa at the external cervical os while avoiding, as far as possible, direct contact with vaginal secretions and spilling from the vagina. Unfortunately, artificial insemination for oligozoospermia has not been very successful.

Asthenospermia

Progressive motility is crucial for the fertilizing capacity of sperm cells. Reduced motility has more often been associated with infertility than reduced sperm concentration or increased percentage of abnormally configured sperm cells (Glezerman et al. 1980). Asthenospermia is a condition in which less than 50% of the sperm cells move progressively.

Artificial insemination with asthenospermic semen seems to offer no distinct advantage over the natural insemination process. However, if semen is treated successfully in vitro by medical or mechanical means, subsequent insemination may be employed.

Impotence

In impotent men, AIH is contraindicated until sexual therapy has been tried and proven unsuccessful. Even then, AIH should be instituted only after marriage counseling has been provided.

In cases of organic impotence (paraplegics, diabetic neuropathy) in whom causal treatment has been ineffective, AIH is the treatment of choice.

Anejaculation may have a variety of causes (endocrine, anatomic, psychogenic). Following evaluation and treatment, some patients may still require artificial procedures to obtain semen for insemination. Electro-vibration may be used for this purpose (Glezerman and Lunenfeld, 1976).

Retrograde Ejaculation

Retrograde ejaculation, often mistakenly described as anejaculation, is an indication for AIH. In this condition, the semen is ejected backward into the bladder, rather than forward through the urethra. The diagnosis of retrograde ejaculation is made by observing sperm cells in the postcoital urine. In these patients, fertility can be achieved by restoration of antegrade ejaculation using alpha-sympaticomimetic agents (Virupannavar and Tomera, 1982) or through efforts to regain viable and fertile sperm from the urinary bladder after sexual intercourse or masturbation, with subsequent artificial insemination. In order to avoid possible damage to the sperm cells by contact with the urine, its acidity is neutralized by administering alkalizing agents prior to intercourse. When the urine is received, it is washed with nutrient solutions (Eagle's solution, Ringer's solution, etc.) and centrifuged and the female partner is inseminated with the sediment (Glezerman et al. 1976b). Scammell et al. (1982) have used human serum albumin for the suspension of retrieved semen and subsequent successful AIH.

Female Factors

Vaginism

Intravaginal AIH is very effective in these cases. However, we feel that fertility-promoting therapy in couples with a sexual problem such as vaginism should be postponed until adequate psycho-sexual treatment has been provided.

Cervical Factor

It is generally accepted that poor function of the uterine cervix may impede sperm transport resulting in infertility (see Chapter 8). If the uterine cervix impedes sperm transport, then artificial bypassing of the uterine cervix may solve the problem (intrauterine AIH).

The split insemination technique is uniquely suited for intrauterine insemination. In cases of so-called immunological infertility – the presence of anti-sperm antibodies on either sperm cells or within the cervical mucus – intrauterine insemination using the first split fraction may also be effective.

Intrauterine insemination using either the split portion or using washed semen has produced rather satisfactory results (Table 14–1).

TABLE 14-1. Pregnancies following Intrauterine Inseminations

Authors (Year)	No. of Patients	Pregnancies
Balmaceda et al. (1984)	20	10 (50 %)
Glezerman et al. (1984)	25	13 (52 %)
Kerin et al. (1984)	39	8 (21 %)
Sher et al. (1984)	51	19 (37 %)

Contraindications for Artificial Homologous Insemination

Absolute or relative contraindications for AIH are present:

1. whenever pregnancy is contraindicated for medical or psychological reasons.
2. in cases of incompatibilities (such as the Rh factor).
3. if either of the partners carries a hereditary disease.
4. in cases of severe systemic diseases in either of the partners (such as lues, severe forms of diabetes mellitus, etc.).
5. when cytostatic or immunosuppressive treatment has been applied recently (up to 1 year before attempted AIH).
6. when either partner has received X-ray therapy (up to 4 months before attempted AIH).
7. in cases of acute genital infection is present in either partner.

Results of Artificial Homologous Insemination

The success rate of artificial homologous insemination varies widely with its indication, and ensuing pregnancies are not always easily attributable to the AIH procedure. Generally, comparing data is difficult, since multifactorial infertility is often treated by AIH, equivocal indications are sometimes present, and data are not always completely reported (Glezerman, 1982). Artificial homologous insemination in cases of severe oligozoospermia (less than 10 million sperm cells per ml), asthenospermia (less than 50% motility) or teratospermia (less than 50% normally configured sperm cells) has rarely produced pregnancy rates in a range which might be considered clearly beyond the rate of chance. However, if the quality of semen is improved before insemination, treatment success is considerably higher. We have employed AIH in 21 patients in whom reduced sperm concentration was due to high seminal volume (dilution oligozoospermia). The mean spermatozoal concentration was 12.4 million per ml (S.E. 4.8 million/ml). The mean volume of seminal fluid was 4.9 ml (S.E. 1.1 ml). In 11 cases the first ejaculatory spurt contained at least twice as many sperm cells per ml than the following spurts. These males were advised to perform "split" intercourse during the periovulatory period. Five of these 11 patients reported difficulties in performing split intercourse and "split AIH" was applied, using the first ejaculatory spurt. The wives of all 11 men conceived within 7 months. In ten males, the first ejaculatory spurt contained less than twice the spermatozoal concentration of the following spurts. Split intercourse or split AIH resulted in five pregnancies in this group. Thus, the total pregnancy rate in these 21 couples was 76.2% following either split intercourse or split AIH.

If no pregnancy ensues following six consecutive AIH cycles, the couple should be reevaluated.

Artificial insemination is not an innocuous procedure and its value must be weighed carefully against possible adverse effects. Whenever AIH is employed, the danger of a mechanization of the sexual relationship should be taken into consideration. The couple may perceive the process of AIH not as a purely medical procedure, but rather as a corrective measure for performance inability. Consequently, the archaic perception of the connection between sexuality and procreation may surface and guilt feelings, subconscious accusations, and injury to the ego of the "responsible" partner may ensue. It is not rare to see previously ovulatory cycles turn anovulatory as soon as treatment with AIH is started, and various degrees of impaired sexual response may occur in either partner (Beck, 1976). For the male who has to produce an ejaculate on demand at a given time, performance coercion is even more evident and presents the most immediate psychological drawback to AIH. The resulting continuous stress situation for the couple and cumulative month-to-month failures exert a tremendous emotional effect on the marriage in general and the sexual relationship in particular. Considering this background, the decision for AIH has to be made very carefully.

ARTIFICIAL DONOR INSEMINATION (AID)

Artificial insemination using donor semen (AID) is probably the most effective tool to provide a barren couple with the desired child if fertilization by the husband is either not feasible or not desirable. It has been estimated that nearly 1 million people owe their existence to AID and between 20,000 to 40,000 children are born annually worldwide as a result of AID.

Indications for AID

The most common indication is absolute male sterility, such as in cases of Klinefelter's syndrome, hypergonadotropic hypogonadism, and therapy-resistant azoospermia. Long-standing infertility in couples in which any degree of oligozoospermia, teratospermia, or asthenospermia of the husband's semen remains resistant to therapy is the next most common indication. Inheritable diseases in the husband's line (e.g., Tay-Sachs disease, juvenile diabetes, Huntington's chorea, etc.) are also indications for AID. So are incompatibilities, such as those concerning the Rh factor when the female partner is sensitized. Finally, in long-standing infertility with no apparent etiology when the female partner is approaching the end of her reproductive years, AID may be considered as a last measure.

Although sperm banks have existed worldwide for a long time, fresh donor semen has usually been preferred by clinicians, who claim better results than with frozen semen. Using patients as their own controls, Richter et al. (1984) have observed that fresh semen is more than three times as likely to induce pregnancy as frozen semen. On the other hand, in a prospective randomized study (Iddenden et al. 1985), no difference in pregnancy rates could be observed between the two modalities. Sherman (1986) has repeatedly stressed the superiority of frozen semen versus fresh semen for AID. Lately, the danger of AIDS transmission has made the use of fresh semen dangerous and State Regulations will most probably prohibit the use of fresh semen in the near future. Last but not least, the use of sperm banks makes the donor artificial insemination program much easier. Although pregnancy rates when frozen semen is used are still somewhat lower than when fresh semen is employed, there are many advantages which probably will cause the disappearance of AID services using fresh semen:
1. Logistics of donor organization are much easier and cheaper.
2. Matching is easier when there is a large number of different semen specimens to choose from.
3. Frozen semen can be exchanged or transported over a large geographical area, minimizing the likelihood of inbreeding by the offspring of a donor.
4. Couples can be given the opportunity of multiple pregnancies from the same donor.
5. Frozen semen is cheaper, since one ejaculate can be used for several inseminations.
6. The risk of AIDS transmission is negligible if current quarantine regulations are followed.

Results of AID

Pregnancy rates with AID are excellent and compare favorably even with spontaneous pregnancy rates in fertile couples after discontinuation of contraception (Table 14-2).

Pregnancy outcome following AID is similar to that in the general population. Table 14-3 presents data obtained in a study of 440 cases treated by AID (Glezerman and Potashnik, 1988).

Using fresh donor semen, more than 70% of treated women will eventually become pregnant, the specific insemination technique playing no significant role (Table 14-4).

TABLE 14-2. Accumulative Pregnancy Rates following Artificial Donor Insemination (AID) and Spontaneous Pregnancy Rates in Women following Discontinuation of Contraception (observed). Data of AID from Glezerman (1981); data of Spontaneous Pregnancy Rates following Discontinuation of Contraception from Tietze (1968)

No. of Cycle	No. of Women		No. of Pregnancies		Cumulative Pregnancy Rate	
	AID	observed	AID	observed	AID	observed
1	270	611	69	199	30.0%	32.6%
2	201	412	57	103	54.7%	49.4%
3	144	309	34	64	69.5%	59.9%
4	110	245	13	36	75.2%	65.8%
5	97	197	11	33	80.0%	71.5%
6	81	157	15	30	86.5%	77.0%
7	64	118	6	18	89.1%	80.5%
8	53	95	6	13	91.7%	83.2%
9	43	77	4	9	93.4%	85.1%
10	37	63	2	10	94.3%	87.5%
11	31	48	4	3	96.0%	88.3%
12	21	43	2	–	96.9%	88.3%
Later	18	38	7	9		
Total			230	257		

TABLE 14-3. Pregnancy Outcome in 371 Pregnancies obtained by AID (from: Glezerman and Potashnik, 1988)

Take home babies	287
Delivery of normal infants	275 (82.3%)
Perinatal deaths	5 (1.5%)
Ectopic pregnancies	2 (0.6%)
Spontaneous abortions	51 (15.6%)
Artificial abortions	1
Pregnant and lost for follow-up	8
Lost for follow-up	29
Total	371
Multiple pregnancy rate	12/371 = 3.2%

TABLE 14-4. Pregnancy Rates with AID using Fresh Semen

Authors (Year)	Patients	Rate	Method
Behrmann (1959)	168	75.0%	?
Haman (1959)	399	76.0%	Pericervical
Murphy and Torrano (1966)	112	68.0%	Intracervical
Warner (1974)	320	72.0%	Pericervical
Whitelaw (1974)	1000	76.6%	Cervical, cap
Chong and Taymor (1975)	107	72.0%	Intracervical, vaginal
Goss (1975)	113	79.6%	Intracervical, vaginal
Dixon and Buttram (1976)	176	44.9%	Pericervical
Sulewski et al. (1978)	121	37.0%	Intracervical, cap
Corson (1980)	137	68.6%	Intracervical, vaginal
Aiman (1982)	105	74.3%	?
Glezerman and Potashnik (1988)	440	84.9%	Pericervical, cap

An analysis of the cumulative distribution of 1,909 pregnancies according to the number of insemination cycles reveals that almost 53% of those women who eventually conceive do so within the first three cycles of treatment, and nearly 80% within six cycles (Table 14-5). A fair chance for treatment success should thus be based on at least six ovulatory cycles, following which the wife should be reevaluated and continuation of the AID program discussed with both partners.

TABLE 14-5. Pregnancy Rates (P.R.) relative to Number of Insemination Cycles (AID) with Fresh Semen

Authors (Year)	Pregnancies	P.R.* 3 Cycles	following 6 Cycles
Behrmann (1959)	126	59.0%	86.0%
Haman (1959)	303	67.0%	87.0%
Murphy and Torrano (1966)	76	62.0%	92.0%
Whitelaw (1974)	766	35.4%	69.5%
Chong and Taymor (1975)	77	73.0%	95.0%
Dixon and Buttram (1976)	79	72.1%	95.0%
Sulewski et al. (1978)	45	69.8%	88.9%
Corson (1980)	94	68.0%	83.0%
Aiman (1982)	78	82.1%	99.0%
Glezerman and Potashnik (1988)	371	69.5%	86.8%

* Pregnancy Rate = Percentage of total number of all pregnancies

TREATMENT OF MALE INFERTILITY AND ASSISTED REPRODUCTION

Our knowledge about the physiology and pathophysiology of the male reproductive function has dramatically improved during the last two decades. Most clinicians agree that the treatment of varicocele, split intercourse, and in vitro treatment of semen with subsequent artificial insemination have merits in the treatment of male infertility. However, no major breakthrough has occurred as far as the medical treatment of male infertility is concerned. The group of men who will benefit from treatment with gonadotropins is extremely small and virtually all other forms of medical treatment have remained rather empirical. For many years, artificial donor insemination has been the main tool in assisted reproduction. It is a convenient bypass of the problematics of treatment of male infertility. The past decade has seen tremendous advances in other areas of assisted reproduction. In vitro fertilization (IVF), embryo transfer (ET), Gamete Intra-Fallopian Transfer (GIFT), Zygote Intra-Fallopian Tube Transfer (ZIFT), Tubal Embryo Transfer (TET), and the micromanipulation of gametes are some of new exiting areas. The infertile male has his share in the benefits these new techniques provide for the infertile couple. Male infertility is now regarded as one indication for IVF (Cohen et al. 1985; Englert et al. 1987; Gibbons, 1987). Van der Merwe et al. (1989a) have successfully used GIFT with washed spermatozoa in men with sperm autoimmunity. Applying GIFT, the same group (Van der Merwe et al. 1989b) has demonstrated a pregnancy rate of 25% in couples in which the male partner suffered from severe teratospermia with only 4–14% normal forms.

Balmaceda et al. (1989) have reported positive results with TET in severely oligozoospermic men in whom GIFT had not been effective. TET has also been successfully applied in conditions previously considered untreatable, like obstructive azoospermia in cases of congenital absence of the vas deferens (Asch et al. 1989). In cases of neck or tail anomalies, microinjection of sperm nuclei into the ooplasm may be a potential treatment in the future (Sinosich et al. 1989).

Treatment of infertility, male or female, may be a tedious and time-consuming task. However, the growing knowledge of the physiology of reproduction and the greater availability of effective fertility-promoting agents make this challenge easier to meet.

References

References

A

Abylholm T (1981): An andrological study of 51 fertile men. Int. J. Androl. 4: 646.

Adashi EY, Rosnick CE, D'Ercole J, Svoboda ME, van Wyk JJ (1985): Insulin-like growth factors as intraovarian regulators of granulosa cell growth and function. Endocr. Rev. 6:400.

Aiman J (1982): Factors affecting the success of donor insemination. Fertil. Steril. 37: 94.

Ainmelk Y, Belisle S, Carmel M, Tetreault JP (1987): Tamoxifen citrate therapy in male infertility. Fertil. Steril. 48:113.

Aksu MF (1982): Epimestrol and clomiphene in resistant anovulation. In: Abstracts of 10th World Congress of Gynecology and Obstetrics, San Francisco, October 1982, p. 318.

D'Ambrogio G, Garutti C, Golinelli S, Kicivic PM, Genazzani AR (1987): Effects of epimestrol on LH secretion in polycystic ovary (PCO). In: AR Genazzani, A Volpe, F Facchinetti (eds), Proceedings of the 1st International Congress on Gynecological Endocrinology

Amelar RD, Dubin L (1975a): Commentary on epididymal vasostomy, vasovasostomy and testicular biopsy. In: M Boedecker (ed): Current operative urology. Harper & Row, New York, pp. 1181.

Amelar RD, Dubin L (1975b): A new method of promoting fertility. Obstet. and Gynecol. 45: 57.

Amelar RD, Dubin L, Walsh PC (1977): Male Infertility. Saunders, Philadelphia, London, Toronto.

Arbatti NJ, Sheth AR (1987): Measurement of inhibin by immunoassays and receptor assay. In: AR Sheth (ed), Inhibins: Isolation, estimation and physiology, Vol I. CRC press, Boca Raton, pp. 119.

Argonz J, Del Castillo EB (1953): A syndrome characterized by estrogenic insufficiency, galactorrhea and decreased urinary gonadotropin. J. Clin. Endocr. 13: 79.

Arimura A, Schally AV (1970): Progesterone suppression of LH releasing hormone induced stimulation of LH in rats. Endocrinology 87: 653.

Armstrong DT, Kraemer MA, Hixon JE (1975): Metabolism of progesterone by rat ovarian tissue: influence of pregnant mare serum gonadotropin and prolactin. Biol. Reprod. 12: 599.

Armstrong DT, Papkoff H (1976): Stimulation of aromatization of exogenous and endogenous androgens in ovaries of hypophysectomized rats in vivo by follicle stimulatory hormone. Endocrinology 99: 1144.

Arver S (1980): Zinc and zinc ligands in human seminal plasma. Part I: Methodological aspects and normal findings. Int. J. Androl. 3: 629.

Asch R, Ord T, Balmaceda J, Patrizio P, Marello E, Silber S (1989): Infertility due to congenital absence of the vas deferens: Results of a new treatment based on epididymal sperm retrieval, in vitro fertilization and tubal embryo tranfer. Presented at the VI World Congress of In Vitro Fertilization and Alternative Assisted Reproduction, Jerusalem, Israel.

Aubert ML, Kreuter R, Syzoneko PC (1988): Mechanism of action of GnRH and GnRH analogues in sexual maturation and function. Gynecological Endocrinology, 2 (Suppl. 1): 35.

Aulitzky W, Frick J (1985): Pulsatile LHRH-treatment in 2 men with idiopathic hypogonadotropic hypogonadism and 2 men with delayed puberty (constitutional delay). J. Androl. 6 (2. Suppl): 91.

Australian Department of Health (ADH), Canberra, Australia (1981): Computer print out, The human pituitary advisory committee, by courtesy of Prof. R. Shearman. Int. J. Androl. 4: 646.

B

Badano AR, Arcangeli OA, Mirkin A, Miechi H, Rodriguez A, Turner D, Aparicio N, Figueroa Casas PR (1977): La bromocriptina en el tratamiento del sindorome de amenorrea e hiperprolactinemia. Obstetricia y Ginecologia Latinamericana 35: 325.

Bahamondes L, Abdelmassih R, Dachs JN (1979): Survey of 185 sperm analyses of fertile men in an infertility service. Int. J. Androl. 2: 526.

Bailer P, Gips H, Aauskolb R, et al. (1980): Serumkonzentrationsverhalten vor Östradiol-17 Beta und Progesterone bei durch Clomiphen überstimulierten Ovarien. Geburtsh. Frauenheilk. 40: 72.

Baker HWG, Straffon WGE, Murphy G, Davidson A, Burger HG, De Kretser DM (1979): Prostatitis and male infertility: A pilot study. Possible increase in sperm motility with antibacterial chemotherapy. Int. J. Androl. 2: 193.

Balmaceda JP, Schenken RS, Ellsworth LR, Arana JB, Martin B, Asch RH, Burgos L (1984): Intrauterine insemination with washed sperm as treatment for infertility. Fertil. Steril. 42: 322.

Balmaceda JP, Rehomi J, Ord T, Patrizio P, Asch RH (1989): Tubal embryo transfer: Results in cases of oligozoospermia and failed GIFT. Presented at the VI World Congress of In Vitro Fertilization and Alternative Assisted Reproduction, Jerusalem, Israel.

Bandivdekar AH, Vijayalak-Shami S, Moodbidri SS, Sheth AR (1982): Low molecular weight inhibin from sheep, human, rat and chicken testes. J. Androl. 3: 140.

Bandivdekar AH, Moodbidri SS, Sheth AR (1984): FSH receptor binding inhibity activity associated with low molecular weight inhibin from sheep, human, rat and chicken. Experientia 40: 994.

Barbieri RL, Ryan KJ (1983): Bromocriptine: endocrine pharmacology and therapeutic applications. Fertil. Steril. 39: 727.

Barbieri RL, Smith S, Ryan KJ (1988): The role of hyperinsulinemia in the pathogenesis of ovarian hyperandrogenism. Fertil. Steril. 50: 197.

Bardin CW, Shaha C, Mather J, Salomon Y, Margioris AN, Liotta AS, Gerendai I, Chen CL, Krieger DT (1984): Ann. N. Y. Acad. Sci. 438: 346–364.

Barnea ER, Arronet GH, Weissenberg R, Lunenfeld B (1980): Studies on polyspermia. Int. J. Fertil. 25: 303.

Bartak V (1974): Behandlungsverfahren bei männlicher Infertilität. Z. Hautkrankh. 49: 889.

Bartoov B, Eltes F, Langsam J, Snyder M, Fisher J (1982): Ultrastructural studies in morphological assessment of human spermatozoa. Int. J. Androl. Suppl. 5: 81.

Basseti M, Spada A, Pezzo G, et al. (1984): Bromocriptine treatment reduces the cell size in human macroprolactinomas: A morphometric study. J. Clin. Endocrinol. Metab. 58: 268.

Bauminger S, Lindner HR (1975): Periovulatory changes prostaglandin formation and their control. Prostaglandins 9: 737.

Beck WW (1976): A critical look at the legal, ethical and technical aspects of artificial insemination. Fertil. Steril. 27: 1.

Beers WH, Strickland S, Reich E (1975): Ovarian plasminogen activator: relationing to ovulation and hormonal regulation. Cell 6: 387.

Behrman SJ (1959): Artificial insemination. Fertil. Steril. 10: 248.

Behrman SJ (1968): The immune response and infertility: Experimental evidence. In: Progress in Infertility. SJ Behrman and RW Kistner (eds.), Little, Brown Co, Boston, pp. 675–699.

Belchetz PE, Plant TM, Nakai Y, et al. (1978): Hypophysial responses to continuous and intermittent delivery of hypothalamic gonadotropin-releasing hormone. Science. 202: 631.

Ben-Jonathan N, Nicul RS, Porter JJ (1973): Superfusion of hemipituitaries with portal blood. Part I: LRF secretion in castrated and diestrous rats. Endocrinology 93: 497–503.

Bennink HJ (1979): Intermittent bromocriptine treatment for the induction of ovulation in hyperprolactinemic patients. Fertil. Steril. 31 (3): 267–272.

Ben-Nun I, Lunenfeld B, Ben Aderet N (1984): Prevention de la luteinisation premature du follicule par hyperprolactinemie iatrogene volontaire au cours des traitements par HMG hormons. Reprod. Met. 5: 54–57.

Benveniste R, Helman JD, Orth ON et al. (1979): Circulating big human prolactin: Conversion to small human prolactin by reduction of disulfide bonds. J. Clin. Endocrinol. Metab. 48: 883.

Berezin M, Lunenfeld B (1988): Long-Term Follow-Up of Patients with Prolactinoma. 3rd European Workshop on Pituitary Adenomas (Abstract). Amsterdam, Holland.

Berg D, Mickan H, Michael S et al. (1983): Ovulation and pregnancy after pulsatile administration of gonadotropin releasing hormone. Arch. Gynecol. 233: 205.

Berger M (1972): Behandlung der Sterilität mit Cyclofenil. Schweiz. Gynäk. Geburtsh. 3: 209.

Bergh T, Nillius SJ, Wide L (1978): Clinical course and outcome of pregnancies in amenorrheic women with hyperprolactinemia and pituitary tumors. Br. Med. J. 1: 875.

Bergh T, Nillius JS, Wide L (1978b): Bromocriptine treatment of 42 hyperprolactinemic women with secondary amenorrhea. Acta Endocrinol. 78: 435.

Bernstein D, Glezerman M, Zejdel L, Insler V (1977): Quantitative study of the number and size of cervical crypts. In: The uterine cervix in reproduction, V Insler and G Bettendorf (eds.), Georg Thieme Publishers, Stuttgart, pp. 14–21.

Bettendorf G, Apostolakis M, Voigt KD (1961): Darstellung hochaktiver Gonadotropinfraktionen aus menschlichen Hypophysen und deren Anwendung beim Menschen. Proc. Internatl. Fed. Gynecol. Obstet. Vienna. p. 76.

Bettendorf G (1966): Ovarian stimulation in hypophysectomized patients by human gonadotropins. Proc. 5th World Congress on Fertility and Sterility. Excerpta 133: 53–54.

Bettendorf G, Braendle W, Sprotte Ch, Weise Ch and Zimmermann R (1981a): Overall results of gonadotropin therapy. In: Advances in diagnosis and treatment of infertility, V. Insler and G. Bettendorf (eds.), Elsevier North Holland, New York, p. 21.

Bettendorf G, Brendle W, Weise Ch, Poels W (1981b): Effect of gonadotropin treatment during inhibited pituitary function. In: Advances in diagnosis and treatment of infertility, V Insler and G Bettendorf (eds), Elsevier North Holland, New York, p. 43.

Bettendorf G, Braendle W, Lichtenberg V, Lindner UKE (1988): Pharmacologic hypogonadotropism – an advantage for gonadotropin stimulation. Gynecological Endocrinology, 2 (Suppl.1): 66.

Bicsak TA, Vale W, Vaughan J, Tucker EM, Cappel S, Hsue AJW (1987): Hormonal regulation of inhibin production by Sertoli cells. Mol. Cell. Endocrinol. 49: 211.

Bhushana Rao KSP, Masson PL (1977): Structure of cervical mucin. In: The uterine cervix in reproduction, V Insler and G Bettendorf (eds), Georg Thieme Publishers, Stuttgart, pp. 63–67.

Black WP, Govan ADT (1972): Laparoscopy and ovarian biopsy for the assessment of secondary amenorrhea. Am. J. Obstet. Gynecol. 114: 739.

Blackwell RE, Bradley EL, Kline LB et al. (1983): Comparison of dopamine agonists in the treatment of hyperprolactinemic syndromes: a multicenter study. Fertil. Steril. 39: 744.

Blankstein J, Mashiach S, Lunenfeld B (1986): Ovulation Induction and In Vitro Fertilization. Chicago: Year Book, 1986.

Blom E (1950): A one-minute live-dead sperm stain by means of eosin nigrosin. Fertil. Steril. 1: 176.

Blumenfeld Z, Lunenfeld B (1989): The potentiating effect of growth hormone on follicle stimulation with human menopausal gonadotropins in a panhypopituitary patient. Fertil. Steril. 52: 328–331.

Bogdanove EM (1964): The role of the brain in the regulation of gonadotropin secretion. Vitam. and Horm. (New York) 22: 206.

Bohnet HG, Dahlen HG, Wultke W et al. (1976): Hyperprolactinemic anovulatory syndrome. J. Clin. Endocrinol. 42: 132.

Bohnet HG, Hanker JP, Horowski R et al. (1979): Suppression of prolactin secretion by lisuride throughout the menstrual cycle and in hyperprolactinemic menstrual disorders. Acta Endocrinol. 92: 8.

Bohnet HG, Hilland U, Hanker JP, Schneider HPG (1981): Treatment of normoprolactinemic corpus luteum insufficiency with epimestrol. Arch. Gynecol. 232: 632–633.

Bonati P (1974): Recent progress in productive endocrinology. Academic Press, London, New York.

Boonsaeng V (1981): A simple method to measure the liquefication rate of human semen. Andrologia, 13: 342.

Borgman V, Hardt W, Schmidt-Gollwitzer M, Adenauer H, Nagel R (1982): Sustained suppression of testosterone production by the luteinizing hormone-releasing hormone agonist, Buserelin, in patients with advanced prostate carcinoma. Lancet 1: 1097.

Boyar R, Finkelstein JW, Kapen S et al. (1975): Twenty-four hour prolactin secretory pattern during pregnancy. J. Clin. Endocrinol. Metab. 40: 1117.

Breckwoldt M, Neulen J, Wieacker P, Schillinger H (1988): Induction of ovulation by combined GnRH/hMG/hCG treatment. Internatl. Symposium on GnRH analogues in cancer and human reproduction, Geneva, Switzerland, Abstr. 058.

Brinton LA, Hoover R, Fraumeni JF Jr. (1983): Reproductive factors in the aetiology of breast cancer. Br. J. Cancer 47: 757.

Brooks A, Keel BS (1979): The semen analysis: An important diagnostic evaluation. Lab. Med. 10: 686.

Brosens I, Cornillie F (1988): Is there a rationale for GnRH analogues therapy in endometriosis? Gynecological Endocrinology 2 (Suppl. 1): 28.

Brotherton J (1979): Estimation of number, mean size and size contribution of human spermatozoa using a coulter counter. J. Reprod. Fertil. 35: 626.

Broun T, Sepsenwol S (1974): Stimulation of 14-C cyclic AMP accumulation by FSH and LH in testis from mature rats. Endocr. 94: 1028.

Brown JS, MacLeod J, Hotchkiss RS (1968): The results of varicocelectomy in subfertile men. Exhibit. Am. Fert. Soc.

Brown JB (1986): Gonadotropins. In: V Insler & B Lunenfeld (eds), Infertility: male and female, Churchill Livingstone, London, p. 359.

Buch JP, Lamb DJ, Lipshultz LJ, Smith RG (1988): Partial characterisation of a unique growth factor secreted by human Sertoli cells. Fertil. Steril. 49: 658.

Bulietti C, Cosmo E, E di Naldi S, Tabanelli S, Ciotti P, Montagnani F, Jasonni VM (1986): The use of epimestrol as a priming for the induction of ovulation with clomiphene. Abstracts of 1st International Congress on Gynecological Endocrinology, Madonna di Campiglio, March 1986, Parthenon Publ., p. 200.

Burgus R, Butcher M, Ling N et al. (1971): Structure moleculaire du facteur hypothalamique (LRF) d'origine ovine controlant la secretion de l'hormone gonadotrope hypophysaire de luteinisation (LH). C.R. Acad.Sci.[D] (Paris) 273: 1611.

Butler JK (1970): Oestrone response patterns and clinical results following various pergonal dosage schedules. In: Developments in the pharmacology and clinical uses of human gonadotrophins, JK Butler (ed), G.D. Searle & Co., High Wycombe, England, p. 42.

Butt WR, Kennedy JF (1971): Structure activity relationships of protein and polypeptide hormones. In: M Margoulis, FC Greenwood (eds), Protein and Polypeptide Hormones. Excerpta Medica, Amsterdam, p. 115.

Buvat J, Gauthier A, Ardaens K, Buvat Herbaut M, Lemaire A (1982): The effects of tamoxiphen on the hormones and the sperm in 80 oligospermic and asthenospermic men. J. Gynecol. Obstet. Biol. Reprod. 11: 407.

C

Cabau A, Bessis R (1981): Monitoring of ovulation induction with human menopausal gonadotropin and human chorionic gonadotropin by ultrasound. Fertil. Steril. 36: 178.

Calamera JC, Vilar O (1979): Comparative study of sperm morphology with three different staining procedures. Andrologia 11: 255.

Calkins JH, Sigel MM, Nankin HR, Lin T (1988): Interleukin-1 inhibits Leydig cel steroidogenesis in primary culture. Endocrinology 123: 1605.

Callaghan JT, Clearly RE, Crabtree R et al. (1981): Clinical response of patients with galactorrhea to pergolide, a potent long-acting dopaminergic ergot derivative. Life Sciences 28: 95.

Carlborg L, Johansson EDB, Gemzell C (1969): Sialic acid and sperm penetration of cervical mucus in relation to total urinary estrogen excretion and plasma progesterone levels in ovulatory women. Acta Endocr. (Copenhagen) 62: 721.

Carmel PW, Araki S, Ferin M (1976): Pituitary stalk portal blood collection in rhesus monkeys: Evidence for pulsatile release of gonadotropin releasing hormone (GnRH). Endocrinology 99: 243.

Caron GM, Beaulieu M, Raymond V et al. (1978): Dopaminergic receptors in the anterior pituitary gland. J. Biol. Chem. 253: 2244.

Casillas ER (1973): Accumulation of carnitine by bovine spermatozoa during maturation in the epididymus. J. Biol. Chem. 248: 8227.

Caspi E, Levin S, Bukovsky J, Weintraub Z (1974): Induction of pregnancy with human gonadotropins after clomiphene failure in menstruating ovulatory infertility patients. Isr. J. Med. Sci. 10: 249-255.

Caspi E, Ronen J, Schreyer P et al. (1976): Pregnancy and infant outcome after gonadotropin therapy. Br. J. Obstet. Gynaecol. 83: 967.

Cetel NS, Rivier J, Valwe W, Yen SSC (1983): The dynamics of gonadotropin inhibition in women induced by an antagonistic analog of gonadotropin releasing hormone. J. Clin. Endocrinol. Metab. 57: 62.

Channing CP, Kammerman S (1974): Binding of gonadotropins to ovarian cells. J. Clin. Endocrinol. Metab. 7: 493.

Channing CP , Tsafriri A (1974): Regulation of ovulatory processes: ovum maturation, follicular rupture and luteinization. In: Advances in fertility regulation through basic research. WA Sadler and S Segal (eds.), New York: Plenum Press.

Chappel S (1987): The physiological significance of Inhibin. In: AR Sheth (ed), Inhibins: Isolation, estimation and physiology, Vol II. CRC Press, Inc. Boca Raton, Florida, p. 17.

Charny CW, Baum S (1968): Varicocele and infertility. J. Am. Med. Ass. 204: 1165.

Charreau EH, Attramadal A, Torjesen PA, Purvis K, Calandra R, Hansson V (1977): Prolactin binding in rat testis. Specific receptors in interstitial cells. Moll. Cell. Endocrinol. 6: 303.

Chen YDI, Payne AH, Kelch RP (1976): FSH stimulating of Leydig cell function in hypophysectomized immature rats. Proc. Soc. Exp. Biol. Med. 153: 473.

Chilton BS, Nicosia SV, Laufer MR (1980a): Effect of estradiol 17-B on cervical cytodifferentiation and glycoprotein synthesis in ovariectomized rabbit. Biol. Reprod. 23: 667.

Chilton BS, Nicosia SV, Sowinski JM, Wolf DP (1980b): Isolation and characterization of rabbit endocervical cells. J. Cell. Biol. 86: 172.

Chiodini P, Liuzzi A, Cozzi R et al. (1981): Size reduction of macroprolactinomas by bromocriptine or lisuride treatment. J. Clin. Endocrinol. Metab. 53: 737.

Chong AP, Taymor ML (1975): Sixteen years' experience with therapeutic donor insemination. Fertil. Steril. 26: 791.

Chretien FC (1977): Technical problems involved in scanning electron microscope observation of cervical mucus framework. In: The uterine cervix in reproduction, V Insler and G Bettendorf (eds.), Georg Thieme Publishers, Stuttgart, pp. 44-52.

Christensen AK, Mason NR (1976): Comparative ability of seminiferous tubules and interstitial tissue of rat testes to synthesize androgens from progesterone-4 14-C in vitro. Endocrinology 76: 646.

Cockett ATK, Takihara H, Cosentino MJ (1984): The varicocele. Fertil. Steril. 41: 5.

Coelingh-Bennink HJT (1983): Induction of ovulation by pulsatile intravenous administration of LHRH in polycycstic ovarian disease. (Abstract). The 65th Annual Meeting of the Endocrine Society, San Antonio, Texas, June 8-10, 1983.

Cohen J, Edwards R, Fehilly C, Fishel S, Hewitt J, Purdy J, Rowland G, Steptoe P, Webster J (1985): In vitro fertilisation: A treatment for male infertility. Fertil. Steril. 43: 422.

Collier JG, Flower RJ, Stanton SL (1975): Seminal prostaglandins in fertile men. Fertil. Steril. 26: 868.

Contreras P, Generini G, Michelsen H et al. (1981): Hyperprolactinemia and galactorrhea: Spontaneous versus iatrogenic hypothyroidism. J. Clin. Endocrinol. Metab. 53: 1036.

Corenblum B, Sirek AMT, Horvath E et al. (1976a): Human mixed somatotrophic and lactotrophic pituitary adenomas. J. Clin. Endocrinol. Metab. 42: 857.

Corenblum B, Pairaudeal N, Shewchuck AB (1976b): Prolactin hypersecretion and short luteal phase defects. Obstet. Gynecol. 47: 486.

Corenblum B, Hanley DA (1981): Bromocriptine reduction of prolactinema size. Fertil. Steril. 36: 716.

Corenblum B, Taylor PJ (1983): Prolactin in current problems in Obstetrics and Gynecology. Vol. VI no. 6, Year Book Medical Publishers, Inc. Chicago, p. 50.

Corson SL (1980): Factors affecting donor artificial insemination success rates. Fertil. Steril. 33: 415.

Cortes-Prieto J, Rubio Martize M, Pesenti B, Soler Villalobos A, Guzman Clavijo M (1981): Treatment of chronic anovulation and corpus luteum deficiency with epimestrol. Reproduction 5: 49–57.

Crooke AC (1970): Comparison of the effect of pergonal and human pituitary follicle stimulating hormone. In: Developments in the pharmacology and clinical uses of human gonadotrophins, JK Butler (ed.), GD Searle & Co., High Wycombe, England.

Crosignani PG, Ferrari C, Liuzzi A et al. (1982): Treatment of hyperprolactinemic states with different drugs: a study with bromocriptine, metergoline and lisuride. Fertil. Steril. 37: 61.

Crowley WF, McArthur JW (1980): Stimulation of the normal menstrual cycle in Kallman's syndrome by pulsatile administration of luteinizing hormone releasing hormone. J. Clin. Endocrinol. Metab. 51: 173.

Crowley WF, Comite F, Vale W, Rivier J, Loriaux DL, Cutler GB (1981): Therapeutic use of pituitary desensitization with a long-acting LH-RH agonist: a potential new treatment for idiopathic precocious puberty. J. Clin. Endocrinol. Metab. 52: 370.

D

Darmasetiawan MS, Jacoeb TZ, Surjana EJ, Soebijanto S, Rachman IA, Samil RS (1985): Clinical and hormonal profile of anovulatory infertile cases treated with epimestrol (Stimovul). In: Khalid BAK, Ng ML (eds.), Proceedings of the 3rd Congress of endocrinology and diabetes for practicing physicians, Kuala Lumpur, December 1985.

Da Rugna D, Stahel T (1976): Über die Wirkungen von Arginin bei der Behandlung von Fertilitätsstörungen des Mannes. Praxis 65: 481.

Dattatreymurty B, Raghavan VP, Purandare TV, Sheth AR, Rao SS (1975): Synergistic action of prolactin with hCG on rat ventral prostate. J. Reprod. Fert. 44: 555.

Davajan V, Kunitake GM (1969): Fractional in vivo and in vitro examination of postcoital cervical mucus in the human. Fertil. Steril. 20: 197–210.

Davajan V, Nakamura RM and Mishell DR Jr. (1971): A simplified technique for evaluation of the biophysical properties of cervical mucus. Am. J. Obstet. Gynec. 109: 1042–1048.

David G, Jouannet P, Martin Boyce A, Spira A, Schwartz D (1979): Sperm counts in fertile and infertile men. Fertil. Steril. 31: 453.

Davidson JM (1969): In: Frontiers in Neuroendocrinology, WF Ganon, L Martini (eds.), Oxford University Press, p. 343.

Davies J, Woolf RB (1961): Histology and fine structure of the adult human cervix uteri. Clin. Obstet. and Gynec. 6: 265–304.

Davis JS (1960): Hormonal control of plasma and erythrocyte volume of rat uterus. Am. J. Physiol. 199: 841.

Davoren JB, Hsueh AJW (1986): Growth hormone increased ovarian levels of immunoreactive somatomedin c/Insuline-like growth factor I in vivo. Endocrinology 118: 888.

De Almeida M, Herry M, Testart J, Belaisch-Allart J, Frydman R, Jouannet A (1987): In vitro fertilization results from thirteen women with antisperm antibodies. Human Reprod. 29: 309–313.

De Kretser DM, Taft HP, Brown JB, Evans JH, Hudson B (1968): Endocrine and histological studies on oligospermic men treated with human pituitary and chorionic gonadotropin. J. Endocr. 40: 107.

Del Castillo EB, Trabucco A, de la Balze AF (1947): Syndrome produced by absence of the germinal epithelium without impairment of the Sertoli or Leydig cells. J. Clin. Endocrinol. Metab. 7: 493.

Delitola G, Wass JAH, Stubbs WA et al. (1979): The effect of lisuride hydrogen maleate, an ergot derivative, on anterior pituitary hormone secretion in man. Clin. Endocrinol. 11: 1.

Del Pozo E, Varga L, Wyss H, Tolis G, Friesen H, Wenner R, Vetter L, Uetwiler A (1974): Clinical and hormonal response to bromocriptine (CB154) in the galactorrhea syndrome. J. Clin. Endocrinol. Metab. 39: 18–26.

Del Pozo E, Wyss H, Lancranjan I, Obolensky W, Verga L (1976): Prolactin-induced luteal insufficiency and its treatment with bromocriptine: preliminary results. In: Ovulation in the human. PG Crosignani (ed.), Academic Press, New York, p. 297.

Del Pozo E, Flueckiger E, Lancranjan I (1976): Endogenous control of prolactin release and its modification by drugs. In: A Charro, R Fernandez Durango, G Lopez del Campo (eds.), Basic Applications and Clinical Use of Hypothalamic Hormones, Amsterdam, Excerpta Medica, p. 137.

Del Pozo E (1982): Hyperprolactinemia in male Infertility: Treatment with Bromocriptine. In: J Bain, WB Schill, L Schwarzstein (eds.), Treatment of male infertility. Springer Verlag, Berlin Heidelberg New York, p. 71.

Denef C (1981): LHRH stimulates prolactin release from rat pituitary lactotrophs cocultured with a highly purified population of gonadotrophs. Ann. Endocrinol. (Paris), 42: 65.

Derrick FC, Yarbrough W, D'Agostino J (1973): Vasovasostomy: results of questionnaire of members of AUA. J. Urol. 110: 556.

Dierschke DJ, Yamaji FJ, Wick RF, Weiss G, Knobil E (1973): Blockade by progesterone of oestrogen induced LH and FSH release in the rhesus monkey. Endocrinol. 92: 1946.

Dixon RE, Buttram VC (1976): Artificial insemination using donor semen: A review of 171 cases. Fertil. Steril. 27: 130.

Dmowski WP, Ericcson RJ, Broer KH, Carruthers KJ (1980): Use of albumin columns in male infertility. In: JC Emperaire, A Audebert, ESE Hafez (eds.), Homologuous artificial insemination (AIH). Nijoff, The Hague, pp. 84.

Dmowski WP, Radwanska E, Binor Z, Tumon I, Pepping P (1988): GnRH analogues in the management of endometriosis. Gynecological Endocrinology, 2 (Suppl. 1): 29.

Docke F, Dorner G (1965): The mechanism of the induction of ovulation by oestrogens. J. Endocr. 33: 491.

Doehr SA, Moghissi KS (1973): Human and bovine cervical mucus. In: RJ Blandau and K Moghissi (eds.): The biology of the cervix. The University of Chicago Press, Chicago and London, pp. 125–142.

Dorsey JW (1973): Surgical correction of post-vasectomy sterility. J. Urol. 110: 554.

Doughtery KA, Cokett ATK, Urry RL (1976): Caffeine, theophylline and human sperm motility. Fertil. Steril. 27: 541.

Dubin L, Amelar RD (1970): Varicocele size and results of varicocelectomy in selected subfertile men with varicocele. Fertil. Steril. 21: 8.

Dufau LM, Charreau EM, Catt HJ (1973): Characteristics of soluble gonadotropin receptor from the rat testis. J. Biol. Chem. 248: 6973.

Dym M, Fawcett DW (1970): The blood-testes barrier in the rat and the physiological compartmentation of the seminiferous epithelium. Biol. Reprod. 3: 308.

E

Eckstein B, Ravard R (1974): On the mechanism of the onset of puberty: identification and pattern of 5α-androstane-3, 17-diol and its 3α-empimer in peripheral blood of premature female rats. Endocrinology, 94: 224.

Eldridge JC, Dmowski WP, Mahesh VB (1974): Effect of castration in immature rats on serum FSH and LH and of various steroid treatments after castration. Biol. Reprod. 10: 438.

Eliasson R, Hellinga G, Luebcke F, Meyhoefer W, Nierman H, Steeno O, Schirren C (1970): Empfehlungen zur Nomenklatur in der Andrologie. Andrologia 2: 186.

Eliasson R (1977): Semen analysis and laboratory workup. In: ATK Cocket and RL Urry (eds.), Male infertility, Grune and Stratton, New York, San Francisco, London, p. 169.

Eliasson R (1981): Analysis of semen. In: H Burger, D De Kretser (eds.), The testis, Raven Press, New York, p. 381.

Elkind-Hirsch K, Schiff I, Ravnikar V et al. (1982): Determinations of endogenous immunoreactive luteinizing hormone releasing hormone in human plasma. J. Clin. Endocrinol. Metab. 54: 602.

Ellis JD, Williamson JG (1975): Factors influencing the pregnancy and complication rates with human menopausal gonadotropin therapy. Br. J. Obstet. Gynaec. 82: 52–57.

Elstein M (1970): The proteins of cervical mucus and the influence of progestagens. J. Obstet. Gynaec. Brit. Cwlth. 77: 443–456.

Elstein M, Daunter B (1973): Trace elements in cervical mucus. In: M Elstein, R Borth and KS Moghissi (eds.), Cervical mucus in human reproduction, Scriptor, Copenhagen, pp. 122–127.

Elstein M (1974): The cervix and its mucus. Clinics in Obstetrics and Gynaecology 1: 345–368.

Elstein M, Daunter B (1977): The electron microscopy of human cervical mucus in the normal menstrual cycle and the first trimester of pregnancy. In: V Insler and G Bettendorf (eds): The uterine cervix in reproduction, Georg Thieme Publishers, Stuttgart, pp. 52–56.

Emons G (1988): The use of GnRH analogues in ovarian cancer. Gynecological Endocrinology, 2 (Suppl. 1): 48.

Emperaire JC, Gauzere-Soumiriev E, Audebert AJM (1982): Female infertility and donor insemination. Fertil. Steril. 37: 90.

Engel T, Jewelewicz R, Dyrenfurth I (1972): Ovarian hyperstimulation syndrome. Am. J. Obstet. Gynecol. 112: 1052.

Englert Y, Vekemans M, Lejeune B, Van Rysselberge M, Puissant F, Degueldre M, Leroy F (1987): Higher pregnancy rates after in vitro fertilisation and embryo transfer in cases with sperm defects. Fertil. Steril. 48: 254.

Eroschenko VP (1978): Alterations in the testes of the Japanese during and after ingestion of the insecticide Kepone. Toxicol. Appl. Pharmacol. 43: 535.

Eshkol A, Lunenfeld B, Insler V, Homburg R (1975): The effect of sex steroids on pituitary responsiveness to gonadotropin releasing hormone. In: T Schellen (ed.), Releasing factors and gonadotropic hormones in male and female sterility: Radioimmunoassays as diagnostic tools in gynecology and andrology, European Press Medikon, Ghent, Belgium, p. 36–46.

Evans J, Townsend L (1976): The induction of ovulation. Obstet. Gynecol. 125: 321.

F

Falk HC, Kaufman SA (1950): What constitutes a normal semen? Fertil. Steril. 1: 489.

Fand B (1973): The histochemistry of human cervical epithelium. In: RJ Blandau and K

Moghissi (eds.), The biology of the cervix, The University of Chicago Press, Chicago and London, pp. 103–124.

Farris EJ (1949): The number of spermatozoa as an index of fertility in man. A study of 406 semen samples. J. Urol. 61: 1099.

Fawcett DW (1975): Ultrastructure and function of the Sertoli cell. In: DW Hamilton, RO Greep (eds.), Male reproductive system, Am. Phys. Soc., Washington, DC, p. 21.

Feek CM, Sawers JSA, Brown NS et al. (1980): Influence of thyroid status on dopaminergic inhibition of thyrotropin and prolactin secretion: Evidence for an additional feedback mechanism in the control of thyroid hormone secretion. J. Clin. Endocrinol. Metab. 51: 585.

Ferrari C, Paracchi A, Rondena M et al. (1976): Effect of two serotonin antagonists on prolactin and thyrotropin secretion in men. Clin. Endocrinol. 5: 575.

Ferrari C, Reschini E, Peracchi M et al. (1980): Endocrine profile and therapeutic employment of a new prolactin lowering drug, metergoline. Gynecol. Obstet. Invest. 11: 1.

Fiddes JC, Goodman HM (1979): Isolation, cloning and sequence analysis of the cDNA for the alpha-subunit of human chorionic gonadotropin. Nature 281: 351.

Figuerora Casas PR, Arcangeli OA, Arrue Gowland CM, Badano AR, Berli RR, Bonofiglio EC (1970): Effect of clomiphene citrate upon parameters of ovulation in patients selectively operated upon during drug administration. Am. J. Obstet. Gynecol. 106: 828–832.

Fleming R, Carter N, Jamieson ME, Black WP, Coutts JTR (1988): Combined buserelin and exogenous gonadotropins (hMG/hCG) ovulation induction in infertile women with normal menstrual rhythm: results and implications. Gynecological Endocrinology, 2 (Suppl.1): 69.

Flueckiger E, Marko M, Doepfner W, Niederer W (1976): Effects of ergot alkaloids on the hypothalamic pituitary axis. Postgrad. Med. J. (Suppl. 1) 52: 57–61.

Forbes AP, Hennemann PH, Griswold GC, Albright F (1954): Syndrome characterized by galactorrhea, amenorrhea and low urinary FSH. J. Clin. Endocrinol. 14: 265–273.

Forest MG, Lecornu M, Peretti E (1980): Familial male pseudohermaphrodism due to 17–20 desmolase deficiency. In vivo endocrine studies. J. Clin. Endocrinol. Metab. 50: 826.

Forest MG, Roulier R (1982): Kinetics of steroidogenic responses to hCG in relation to age or previous gonadotropin environment: induction of steroidogenic desensitization by pretreatment with hCG in hypogonadotrophic hypogonadic (HH) adult men. Advance mini posters of the Second European Workshop on the Testis, Rotterdam, The Netherlands, p. 9.

Franchi F, Luisi M, Kicovic PM (1978): Long-term study of oral testosterone undecanoate in hypogonadal males. Int. J. Androl. 3: 1.

Franchimont P (1972): Human gonadotropin secretion. J. R. Coll. Physicians, London 6: 283.

Franchimont P (1973a): Regulation des fonctions gonadiques. Bull. Acad. R. Med. Belg. 128: 380.

Frank S, Nabarro JDN, Jacobs HS (1977): Prevalence and presentation of hyperprolactinemia in patients with functionless pituitary tumors. Lancet 1: 778.

Franklin RR, Dukes CD (1964): Antispermatozoal antibody and unexplained infertility. Am. J. Obstet. Gynecol. 89: 6–9.

Franks SD, Horrocks PM, Lynch SS et al. (1981): Treatment of hyperprolactinemia with pergolide mesylate acute effects and preliminary evaluation of long-term treatment. Lancet 2: 659.

Franks S, Jacobs HS (1983): Hyperprolactinemia. Clin. Endocrinol. Metab. 12: 641.

Freund M, Peterson RN (1976): Semen evaluation and infertility. In: ESE Hafez (ed.), Human semen and fertility regulation in man, Mosby, Saint Louis, p. 344.

Friberg J (1974): A simple and sensitive micro-method for demonstration of sperm-agglutinating activity in serum from infertile men and women. Acta Obstet. Gynecol. Scand. (Suppl.) 36: 21.

Friedman AJ, Barbieri RL, Doubilet PM, Fine C, Schiff I (1988): A randomized, double-blind trial of a gonadotropin releasing hormone agonist (Leuprolide) with or without medroxyprogesteroneacetate in the treatment of leiomyomata uteri. Gynecological Endocrinology, 2 (Suppl. 1): 90.

Friedrich ER (1973): The normal morphology and ultrastructure of the cervix. In: RJ Blandau and K Moghissi (eds.), The biology of the cervix, The University of Chicago Press, Chicago and London, pp. 79–102.

Friesen H, Belanger C, Guyda H, Hwang P (1972): The synthesis and secretion of placental lactogen and pituitary prolactin. In: GEW Wolstenholme and J Knight (eds.), Lactogenic hormones, Churchill Livingstone, Edinburgh and London, pp. 83–103.

Frohman LA, Berelowitz M, Gonzales C et al. (1981): Studies of dopaminergic mechanisms in hyperprolactinemic states. In: PG Crosignani, BL Rubin (eds.), Endocrinology of Human Infertility: New Aspects. Serono Clinical Colloquia on Reproduction 2. London, Academic Press, New York, p. 39.

Frommel R (1882): Über puerperale Atrophie des Uterus. Z. Geburtshilfe u. Gynäkologie 7: 305–315.

G

Garcia JE, Jones GS, Acosta AA, Wright G (1983): Human menopausal gonadotropin/ human chorionic gonadotropin in follicular maturation for oocyte aspiration. Phase I. Fertil. Steril. 39: 167.

Gaton E, Zejdel L, Bernstein D, Glezerman M, Czernobilski B, Insler V (1982): The effect of estrogen and gestagen on the mucus production of human endocervical cells: A histochemical study. Fertil. Steril. 38: 580–585.

Geier A, Lunenfeld B, Pariente C, Kotev Emeth S, Kokia E, Shadmi A, Blankstein J (1987): Estrogen receptor binding material in blood of patients following clomiphene citrate administration: Determination by radioreceptor assay. Fertil. Steril. 47: 778–784.

Gellert-Mortimer ST, Clarke GN, Baker HWG, Hyne RV, Johnston WIH (1988): Evaluation of Nycodenz and percoll density gradients for the selection of motile human spermatozoa. Fertil. Steril. 49: 335.

Gemzell CA, Diczfalusy E, Tillinger KG (1958): Clinical effect of human pituitary follicle stimulating hormone (FSH). J. Clin. Endocrinol. 18: 138–148.

Gemzell CA, Diczfalusy E, Tillinger KG (1960): Human pituitary follicle stimulating hormone. 1.: Clinical effect of a partly purified preparation. Ciba Foundation Colloquia on Endocrinology, 13: 191.

Gemzell CA (1970): Recent results of human gonadotropin therapy. In: G Bettendorf and V Insler (eds.), Clinical application of human gonadotropins, Thieme Verlag, Stuttgart, pp. 6–17.

Gemzell CA (1973): Induction of ovulation in patients following removal of pituitary adenoma. Am. J. Obstet. Gynecol. 117: 955–961.

Gemzell CA, Wang CF (1979): Outcome of pregnancy in women with pituitary adenoma. Fertil. Steril. 31: 363.

Genazzani AR, D'Ambrogio G (1986): Epimestrol as modulator of gonadotropin secretion in the treatment of menstrual disorders. In: Abstracts of 1st International Congress on Gynecological Endocrinology, Madonna di Campiglio, March 1986, Parthenon Publ., p. 94.

Giarola A (1974): Effect of Mesterolone on the spermatogenesis of infertile patients. In: RE Mancini and L Martini (eds.), Male fertility and sterility, Academic Press, New York, p. 479.

Gibbons RA, Mattner PE (1971): The chemical and physical characteristics of the cervical secretion and its role in reproductive physiology. In: AI Sherman, C Charles (eds.), Pathways to conception. Thomas, Springfield, Ill., pp. 143–155.

Gibbons RA, Sellwood R (1973): The macromolecular biochemistry of cervical secretions. In: RJ Blandau and K Moghissi (eds.), The biology of the cervix. The University of Chicago and London, pp. 251–265.

Gibbons W (1987): In-vitro fertilization as therapy for male factor infertility. Urol. Clin. North Am. 14: 563.

Gimes R, Toth F (1973): Clinical observations and hormone studies on sterile patients. In: T Haseggawa, M Hayashi, FJG Ebbling and IW Henderson (eds.), Fertility and Sterility. Excerpta Medica, Amsterdam, pp. 663–664.

Glezerman M (1981): 270 cases of artificial donor insemination. Management and results. Fertil. Steril. 35: 180.

Glezerman M (1982): Artificial homologous insemination. In: J Bain, WB Schill, L Schwarzstein (eds.), Treatment of male infertility. Springer Verlag, Berlin – Heidelberg – New York, pp. 295.

Glezerman M (1984): A short historical review and comparative results of surgical treatment for varicocele. In: M Glezerman, EW Jecht, (eds.), Varicocele and male infertility II. Springer Verlag, Berlin – Heidelberg – New York – Tokio, p. 87.

Glezerman M, Lunenfeld B (1976): Zur Therapie der männlichen Anorgasmie. Ein Fallbericht. Akt. Dermat. 2: 167.

Glezerman M, Rakowszyk M, Lunenfeld B, Beer R, Goldman B (1976a): Varicocele in oligospermic patients. Pathophysiology and results after ligation and division of the internal spermic vein. J. Urol. 115: 562.

Glezerman M, Lunenfeld B, Potashnik G, Oelsner G, Beer R (1976b): Retrograde ejaculation: Pathophysiological aspects and report of two successfully treated cases. Fertil. Steril. 27: 796.

Glezerman M, Lunenfeld B, Insler V (1978): Male infertility. In: B Lunenfeld, V Insler: Diagnosis and treatment of functional infertility. Grosse-Verlag, Berlin, p. 114.

Glezerman M, Brook I, Potashnik G, Ben Aderet N, Insler V (1980): Fertility pattern and reported pregnancies in 333 patients referred to male infertility clinics. In: Proceedings of Vth ESCO, Venice. Edizioni Internazionali Gruppo Editoriale Medico, Rome, p. 495.

Glezerman M, Bernstein D, Zakut CH, Misgav N, Insler V (1982): Polyzoospermia. A definite pathological entity. Fertil. Steril. 38: 605.

Glezerman M, Bernstein D, Insler V (1984): The cervical factor of infertility. Int. J. Fertil. 29: 16.

Glezerman M, Jecht EW (1984): Varicocele and male infertility II. Springer Verlag, Berlin – Heidelberg – New York – Tokio

Glezerman M, Potashnik G (1988): Artificial insemination using donor semen. Andrologia 20: 384.

Glezerman M, Bartoov B (1992): Semen analysis. In: V Insler, B Lunenfeld (eds.), Infertility male and female. Churchill-Livingstone, London, in press.

Gnarpe H, Friberg J (1976): The penetration of trimethoprim into seminal fluid and serum. Scand. J. Infect. Dis. Suppl. 8: 50.

Golander A, Hurley T, Barret et al. (1978): Prolactin synthesis by human chorion decidual tissue. A possible source of prolactin in the amniotic fluid. Science, 202: 311.

Goldfarb AF, Schlaff S, Mansi ML (1982): A life table analysis of pregnancy yield in fixed low dose menotropin therapy for patients in whom clomiphene citrate failed to induce ovulation. Fertil. Steril. 37: 629.

Gomez WR, Hall RW, Jain SK, Boots LR (1978): Serum gonadotropin and testosterone levels during loss and recovery of spermatogenesis in rats. Endocr. 93: 800.

Goodman AL, Nixon WE, Johnson DL, Hodgen GD (1977): Regulation of folliculogenesis in the rhesus monkey: selection of the dominant follicle. Endocrinology 100: 155.

Gooren LJG (1986): Long-term safety of the oral androgen testosterone undecanoate. Int. J. Androl. 9: 21.

Gorlitzky GA, Kase N, Speroff L (1978): Ovulation and pregnancy with clomiphene citrate. Obstet. Gynecol. 51: 3.

Goss DA (1975): Current status of artificial insemination with donor semen. Am. J. Obstet. Gynecol. 122: 246.

Gougeon A (1985): Origin and growth of the preovulatory follicle(s) in spontaneous and stimulated cycles. In: J Testart, R Frydman (eds.), Human In Vitro Fertilization, Inserm Symposium No. 24, Elsevier Science Publisher B.V., Amsterdam.

Graf M, Specht A, Distler W (1986): Epimestrol in the treatment of hypothalamic primary amenorrhea. Geburtsh. Frauenheilk. 46: 444–449.

Grandison L, Cavagnini F, Schmid R et al. (1982) : Aminobutyric acid and benzodiazepine binding sites in human anterior pituitary tissue. J. Clin. Endocrinol. Metab. 54: 597.

Greenblatt, RB, Barfield WE, Jungck EC et al. (1961): Induction of ovulation with MRL/41, preliminary report.

Greenblatt RB (1966): Induction of ovulation with clomiphene. In: Ovulation, RB Greenblatt, JB Lippincott Co. (eds.), Philadelphia – Toronto, pp. 134–149.

Greenblatt RB (1968): Experimental studies using clomiphene citrate. In: Progress in Infertility. SJ Behrmann and RW Kistner (eds.), Little, Brown and Co. Boston, pp. 455–466.

Greenblatt RB, Dalla Pria S (1971): Clomiphene in women. In: ChA Joel, Fertility Disturbances in Men and Women, S. Karger A.G., Basel, pp. 541–556.

Griffith RW, Turkalj I, Braun P (1979): Pituitary tumors during pregnancy in mothers treated with bromocriptine. Br. J. Clin. Pharmacol. 7: 393.

Guha K, Vanha-Perttula T (1980): Acid phosphatases of the human testis. Int. J. Androl. 3: 256.

Guillemin R (1978): Peptides in the brain: The new endocrinology of the neuron. Science 202: 390.

Gysler M, March CM, Mishell DR et al. (1982): A decade's experience with an individualized clomiphene treatment regimen including its effect on the postcoital test. Fertil. Steril. 37: 161.

H

Hack M, Lunenfeld B (1978): The influence of hormone induction of ovulation on the fetus and newborn. Pediat. Adolesc. Endocrin. 5: 191.

Hackeloer BJ, Nitschke S, Daume E, Sturm G, Buchholz R (1977): Ultraschalldarstellung von Ovarveränderungen bei Gonadotropinstimulierung. Geburtsh. Frauenheilk. 37: 185.

Hackeloer BJ (1984): The role of ultrasound in female infertility management. Ultrasound in Med. & Biol. 10: 35.

Haesungsharern A, Chulavatnatal M (1973): Stimulation of human spermatozoal motility by caffeine. Fertil. Steril. 24: 66.

Hafez ESE (1973a): The comparative anatomy of the mammalian cervix. In: R Blandau and K Moghissi (eds.), The biology of the cervix, The University of Chicago Press, Chicago and London, pp. 23–56.

Hafez ESE (1973b): Histology and microstructure of the cervical epithelial secretory system. In: M Elstein, KS Moghissi and R Scriptor (eds.), Cervical mucus in human reproduction, Copenhagen, pp. 23–32.

Hafez ESE, Barhanart M, Ludwig H, Lusher J, Joelsson I, Daniel L, Sherman AII, Jordan JA, Wolf H, Stewart WC, Chretien FC (1975): Scanning electron microscopy of human reproduction physiology. Acta Obstet. Gynecol. Scand. Suppl. 40.

Haman SJ (1959): Therapeutic donor insemination. Calif. Med. 90: 130.

Hammerstein J, Schmidt B (1981): Role of epimestrol in induction of ovulation with special reference to 126 pregnancies. In: V Insler, G Bettendorf, KH Geissler (eds.), Advances in diagnosis and treatment of infertility, Elsevier, New York, pp. 131–136.

Hammond MG, Halme J, Talbert LM (1983): Factors affecting the pregnancy rate in clomiphene citrate induction of ovulation. Obstet. Gynecol. 62: 196.

Hanly HG, Harrison RG (1962): The Nature and surgical treatment of varicocele. Br. J. Surg. 56: 64.

Hanson V, Djoseland O, Rousch E, Artamudol A, Torgerson O (1973): An androgen binding protein in the testes cytosol fraction of adult rats. Comparison with androgen binding in the epididymis. Steroids 21: 457–474.

Hardy J (1980): Microsurgical exploration of a normal sella turcica for a microadenoma. In: PJ Derome, CP Jedynake, F Peillon (eds.), Pituitary Adenomas, Asclepios Publishers, France, p. 195.

Harlap S (1976): Ovulation induction and congenital malformations. Lancet 2: 961.

Hawkes RC, Holland GN, Moore WS et al. (1983): The application of NMR imaging to the evaluation of pituitary and juxtasellar tumors. Am. J. Neuroradiol. 4: 221.

Hazout A, Belaisch-Allart J (1986): Prevention des complications de l'induction de l'ovulation par la reduction folliculaire et la reduction embryonnaire. In: J Buvat, J Bringers, Doin Editeurs, Induction et stimulation de l'ovulation, Progres en Gynecologie 1, Paris, p. 156.

Hazum E, Fridkin M, Baram T, Koch Y (1981): Degradation of gonadotropin releasing hormone by anterior pituitary enzymes. F.E.B.S. Lett. 127: 273.

Healy DL, Kovacs GT, Pepperell RJ, Burger HG (1980): A normal cumulative conception rate after human pituitary gonadotropin. Fertil. Steril. 34: 341.

Healy DL, Burger HG (1982): Serum FSH, LH and PRL during the induction of ovulation with exogenous gonadotropins. J. Clin. Endocrinol. Metab.

Healy DL, Lawons SR, Abbott M, Baird DT, Fraser HM (1986): Toward removing uterine fibroids without surgery: subcutaneous infusion of a luteinizing hormone releasing hormone agonist commencing in the luteal phase. J. Clin. Endocrinol. Metab. 63: 619.

Hedon B (1988): Use of GnRH agonists for in vitro fertilization. Gynecological Endocrinology, 2 (Suppl.1): 34.

Heindel JJ, Treinen KA (1989): Physiology of the male reproductive system: Endocrine, paracrine and autocrine regulation. Tox. Pathol. 2: 411–445.

Heite HJ, Wetterauer W (1979): Zur Kenntnis der saueren Phosphatase im Seminalplasma – Bestimmungsmethode und diagnostische Bedeutung. Andrologia 11: 113.

Heller CG, Clermont Y (1964): Kinetics of the germinal epithelium in man. Rec. Progr. Hormone Res. 20: 545.

Hendricks CH: Twinning in relation to birth weight mortality and congenital malformations. Obstet. Gynecol. 27: 47.

Herbert DC (1976): Immunocytochemical evidence that luteinizing hormones (FSH) are present in the same cell in the rhesus monkey pituitary gland. Endocrine, 98: 1554.

Herman V, Kalk WJ, De Moor NG et al. (1981): Serum prolactin after chest wall surgery: Elevated levels after mastectomy. J. Clin. Endocrinol. Metab. 52: 148.

Hewitt J, Cohen J, Krishnaswamy V, Fehilly CB, Steptoe PC, Walters DE (1985): Treatment of idiopathic infertility: insemination with husband's semen or in vitro fertilization? Fertil. Steril. 44: 350–355.

Hilliard J, Schally AV, Sawyer Ch (1971): Progesterone blockade of the ovulatory response to intrapituitary infusion of LHRH in rabbits. J. Endocr. 88: 730.

Hirschel MD, Isahakia MA, Alexander NJ (1984): Characterization of human sperm antigens using monoclonal antibodies. Ann. N.Y. Acad. Sci. 438: 508.

Hodgen GD (1982): The dominant follicle. Fertil. Steril. 38: 281.

Hodgen GD, Goodman AL, Stouffer RL, Williams RF, di Zerega GS, Kreitman OL, Marut EL, Schenken RS (1983): Selection of the dominant follicle and its ovum in the menstrual cycle In: HM Baier and HR Lindner (eds.), Fertilization of the human egg in vitro, Springer Verlag, Berlin, p. 57.

Hoeglund A, Odeblad E (1977): Sperm penetration in cervical mucus: a biophysical and group-theoretical approach. In: V Insler and G Bettendorf (eds.), The uterine cervix in reproduction. Thieme Verlag, Stuttgart, pp. 129–134.

Hokfelt T, Fuxe K (1972): Effects of prolactin and ergot alkaloids on the tubero infundibular dopamine (DA) neurons. Neuroendocrinology 9: 100.

Holcberg G, Kleinman D, Sarov I, Potashnik G, Insler V (1986): Immunoperoxidase assay for detection of special IgG and IgA antibodies to human spermatozoa in infertile women. Int. J. Fertil. 31: 28–39.

Homburg R, Insler V, Lunenfeld B, Eshkol A, Potashnik G: The effects of clomiphene on the pituitary response to gonadotropin releasing hormone. Recent Advances in Human Reproduction, Excerpta Medica.

Homburg R, Eshel A, Abdalla HI, Jacobs HS (1988): Growth hormone facilitates ovulation induction by gonadotropins. Clin. Endocrinol. 29: 113–117.

Hommonai ZT, Paz G, Weiss JN, David MP (1980): Quality of semen obtained from 627 fertile men. Int. J. Androl. 3: 217.

Horowski R, Wachtel H (1976): Direct dopaminergic action of lisuride hydrogen maleate, an ergot derivative, in mice. Europ. J. Pharmacol. 36: 373.

Hotchkiss RS (1970): Infertility in the male. In: MF Campbell, JH Harrison (eds.), Urology. Saunders, Philadelphia, p. 674.

Hotchkiss RS (1972): The role of the urologist in infertile marriage. Bull. N.Y. Acad. Med. 48: 525.

Hudson RW (1988): The endocrinology of varicoceles. Fertil. Steril. 49: 199.

Hulka JF, Omran KF (1969): The uterine cervix as a potential local antibody secretor. Am. J. Obstet. Gynecol. 104: 440–442.

Hull, MGR (1989): Polycystic ovarian disease: clinical aspects and prevalence Research and Clinical Forums 11: 21–30.

Hussa RD (1980): Biosynthesis of human chronic gonadotropin. Endocrine Reviews 1: 268.

Hutson JC, Stocco DM (1981): Peritubular cell influence on the efficiency of androgen-binding protein secretion by Sertoli cells in culture. Endocrinology 108: 1362–1368.

Hwang P, Guyda H, Friesen HG (1972): Purification of human prolactin. J. Biol. Chem. 247: 1955.

I

Iacobelli S, Garcea N, Angeloni C (1971): Biochemistry of cervical mucus; a comparative analysis of the secretion from preovulatory, postovulatory and pregnancy periods. Fertil. Steril. 22: 727–734.

Iddenden DA, Sallam HN, Collins WP (1985): A prospective randomized study comparing fresh semen and cryopreserved semen for artificial insemination by donor. Int. J. Fertil. 30: 54.

Insler V (1977): Evaluation and treatment of cervical mucus diseases leading to infertility. In: DV Parke and M Elstein (eds.), Mucus in health and disease, Plenum Publishing Co., New York, pp. 477–486.

Insler V, Lunenfeld B (1974): Application of human gonadotropins for induction of ovulation In: A Campos da Paz, T Hasegawa, Y Notake and M Hayashi (eds.), Human Reproduction, Igaku Shoin, Tokyo, pp. 25–38.

Insler V, Lunenfeld B (1977): Human gonadotropins. In: EE Philip, J Barnes and M Newton (eds.), Scientific foundation of obstetrics and gynaecology, Heinemann, London, p. 629.

Insler V, Lunenfeld B (1990): Polycystic ovarian disease: a Challenge and controversy. Gynecological Endocrinology 4: 51–69.

Insler V, Lunenfeld B (1991): Pathophysiology of polycystic ovarian disease: new insights. Hum. Reprod. 6: 1025–1029.

Insler V, Potashnik G (1983): Monitoring of follicular development in gonadotropin stimulated cycles. In: HM Beier and HR Lindner (eds.), Fertilization of the human egg in vitro, Springer Verlag, Berlin, p. 111.

Insler V, Melmed H, Mashiah H, Monselise M, Lunenfeld B, Rabau E (1968): Functional classification of patients selected for gonadotropic therapy. Obstet. Gynecol. 32: 620–625.

Insler V, Melmed H, Eden E, Serr DM, Lunenfeld B (1970): Comparison of various methods used in monitoring of gonadotropic therapy. In: G Bettendorf and V Insler (eds),

Clinical application of human gonadotropins, Thieme Verlag, Stuttgart, pp. 87–100.

Insler V, Melmed H, Eden E et al. (1972): The cervical score: A simple semiquantitative method for monitoring of the menstrual cycle. Int. J. Gynaecol. Obstet. 10: 223.

Insler V, Eden E, Serr DM (1973): Induction of ovulation with epimestrol. In: T Hasegawa, M Hayashi, FJG Ebling and JW Henderson (eds.), Fertility and Sterility, Excerpta Medica, Amsterdam, pp. 661–662.

Insler V, Zakut H, Serr DM (1973a): Cycle pattern and pregnancy rate following combined clomiphene estrogen therapy. Obstetrics and Gynecology 41: 602–607.

Insler V, Bernstein D, Glezerman M, Misgav N (1979): Correlation of seminal fluid analysis with mucus penetrating ability of spermatozoa. Fertil. Steril. 32: 316.

Insler V, Glezerman M, Bernstein D, Zejdel L, Misgav N (1981): Cervical crypts and their role in storing spermatozoa. In: V Insler, G Bettendorf, KH Geissler (eds.), Advances in diagnosis and treatment of infertility, Elsevier, North Holland, New York, p. 195.

Insler V, Potashnik G, Glassner M (1981a): Some epidemiological aspects of fertility evaluation. In: V Insler and G Bettendorf (eds.), Advances in diagnosis and treatment of infertility, Elsevier, North Holland, New York, p. 165.

Insler V, Potashnik G, Lunenfeld E, Meizner I, Levy J (1988): Ovulation induction with hMG following down regulation of the hypothalamic pituitary axis by LHRH anlogs. Gynecological Endocrinology, 2 (Suppl. 1): 67.

Isahakia M, Alexander NJ (1984): Vasectomy induced autoimmunity: antisperm and antinuclear autoimmune monoclonal antibodies. Am. J. Reprod. Immunol. 5: 117.

Isojima S, Li TS, Ashitaka Y (1968): Immunologic analysis of sperm-immobilizing factor found in sera of women with unexplained infertility. Am. J. Obstet. Gynecol.

Isomaa V, Parvinen M, Janne OA, Bardin CW (1985): Nuclear androgen receptors in different stages of the seminiferous epithelial cycle and the interstitial tissue of rat testis. Endocrinology 116: 132.

Ivanissevich O, Gregorini H (1918): Uno nuovo operacion para crurar el varicocele. Sem. Med. (B.Airs) 25: 575.

J

Jaeger WH (1988): GnRH analogues in treatment of ovarian carcinoma. Gynecological Endocrinology, 2 (Suppl.)

Jaszczak S (1973): Migration of sperm in the cervix and uterus of nonhuman primates. In: M Elstein, KS Moghissi and R Borth (eds.), Cervical mucus in human reproduction, Scriptor, Copenhagen, pp. 33–34.

Jequier AM (1986): Infertility in the male. Churchill Livingstone, Edinburgh – London – Melbourne – New York.

Jeulin C, Serres C, Jouannet P (1982): The effect of centrifugation, various synthetic media and temperature on the motility and vitality of human spermatozoa. Reprod. Nutr. Dev. 2: 81.

Jeyendran RS, Van der Ven HH, Rosecrans R, Perez-Palaez M, Al Hasani S, Zaneveld LJD (1989): Chemical constituents of human seminal plasma: Relationship to fertility. Andrologia 21: 423.

Jia XC Kalmijin, Hsueh AJW (1985): Growth hormone (GH) augments the FSH induction of LH receptors in cultured granulosa cells. 32nd Annual Meeting of the Society for Gynecologic Investigation. Phoenix, Arizona (Abstract p. 179).

Joel CA (1966): New etiological aspects of habitual abortions and infertility with special reference to the male factor. Fertil. Steril. 17: 374.

Johnsen SG (1970): The human testis. Plenum Press, New York.

Johnsen SG (1972): Gonadotropins. Wily Interscience, New York.

Johnsen OR, Eliasson R, Abdel Kader MM (1974): Effects of caffeine on the motility and metabolism of human spermatozoa. Andrologia 6: 53.

Jordan J, Allen JM (1977): Ultrastructure of the cervical epithelium. In: V Insler and G Bettendorf (eds.), The uterine cervix in reproduction. Georg Thieme Publishers, Stuttgart, pp. 21–35.

Jouannet P, Czyglik F, David G, Mayaux MJ, Moscato ML, Schwartz D (1981): Study of a group of 484 fertile men. Part I: Distribution of semen characteristics. Int. J. Androl. 4: 440.

Jungling ML, Bunge RG (1976): The treatment of spermatogenic arrest with arginine. Fertil. Steril. 27: 282.

Jungmann RA, Hiestand CP, Schweppe JS (1974): Mechanism of action of gonadotropin. IV. Cyclic adenosine monophosphate dependent translocation of ovarian cytoplasmic cyclic adenosine monophosphate binding protein and protein kinase to nuclear acceptor sites. Endocrinology 94: 168–183.

K

Kamberi IA (1975): Brain neurotransmitters and their interaction with the hypothalamo-pituitary-gonadal principles. In: Advances in the biosciences. 15. Schering workshop on actions of estrogenic hormones, pp. 249–266. Pergamon Press, Vieweg.

Kaneko S, Yamagushi J, Kobayashi T, Izuka R (1983): Separation of human X- and Y-bearing sperm using percoll density gradient centrifugation. Fertil. Steril. 40: 661.

Kao LWL, Gunsalas GL, Williams GH, Weisz J (1977): Response of the perfused anterior pituitaries of rats to synthetic gonadotropin releasing hormone: A comparison with hypothalamic extract and demonstration of a role for potassium in the release of luteinizing hormone and follicular stimulating hormone. Endocrinology 101: 1444.

Karten MJ, Rivier JE (1986): Gonadotropin releasing hormone analog design. Structure function studies toward the development of agonists and antagonists: rationale and perspective. Endocr. Rev. 7: 44.

Kastin AJ, Zarate A, Midgley AR, Canales E, Schally AV (1971): Ovulation confirmed by pregnancy after infusion of porcine LHRH. J. Clin. Endocrinol. Metab. 33: 980.

Katzenellenbogen BS, Bhakoo HS, Ferguson ER et al. (1979): Estrogen and antiestrogen action in reproductive tissue and tumors. Recent Prog. Horm. Res. 35: 259.

Kaupila A, Leinonen P, Vihko R et al. (1982): Metoclopramide induced hyperprolactinemia impairs ovarian follicle maturation and corpus luteum function in women. J. Clin. Endocrinol. Metab. 54: 955.

Keiserman WM, Dubin L, Amelar RD (1974): A new type of retrograde ejaculation. Report of three cases. Fertil. Steril. 25: 1071.

Keller PJ (1975a): Ovulationsauslösung mit Clomiphen und Cyclofenil. In: W Obolensky and O Kaeser (eds.), Ovulation und Ovulationsauslösung – Perioperative Probleme. Verlag Hans Huber, Bern, pp. 95–101.

Keller PJ (1975b): Ovulationsauslösung durch Sexualsteroide. In: W Obolensky and O Kaeser (eds.), Ovulation und Ovulationsauslösung – Perioperative Probleme, Verlag Hans Huber, Bern, pp. 88–94.

Kelsey JL (1979): A review of the epidemiology of human breast cancer. Epidemiol. Rev. 1: 74–109.

Kelsey JL, Livolsi VA, Holford TR, Fischer DB, Mostow ED, Schwartz PE, O'Connor T, White C (1982): A case control study of endometrial cancer. Am. J. Epidemiol. 116: 333–342.

Keogh EJ, Mallal SA, Giles PFH (1981): Ovulation induction with intermittent subcutaneous LHRH. Lancet 1: 147.

Kerin JF, Matthews CD, Svigos JM, Makin AE, Symons RG, Smacaton TC (1976): Linear and quantative migration of stored sperm through cervical mucus during the periovular period. Fertil. Steril. 27: 1054–1069.

Kerin JPF, Kirby C, Peek J, Jewffrey R, Warns GM, Matthews CD, Fox LW (1984): Improved conception rate after intrauterine insemination of washed spermatozoa from men with poor quality semen. Lancet March 10, 553.

Keye WR, Ho Yuen B, Knopf RF, Jaffe RB (1976): Amenorrhea, hyperprolactinemia and pituitary enlargement secondary to primary hypothyroidism. Obstet. and Gynecol. 48: 667.

Kistner RW, Smith OW (1961): Observations on the use of nonsteroidal estrogen antagonist Mer-25: Effects in endometrial hyperplasia and Stein-Leventhal syndrome. Fertil. Steril. 12: 121.

Kistner RW (1965): Further observations on the effects of clomiphene citrate in anovulatory females. Am. J. Obstet. Gynecol. 92: 380–411.

Kistner RW (1975): Induction of ovulation with clomiphene citrate. In: SG Behrman and RW Kistner (eds.), Progress in infertility, Little, Brown & Co., Boston, p. 509.

Kistner RW (1976): Sequential use of clomiphene citrate and human menopausal gonadotropin in ovulation induction. Fertil. Steril. 27:72.

Kleinberg DL, Noel GD, Franzi AG (1977): Galactorrhea: a study of 235 cases, including 48 with pituitary tumors. N. Engl. J. Med. 196: 589.

Kleinberg DL, Boyo III AE, Wardlaw A et al. (1983): Pergolide for the treatment of pituitary tumors secreting prolactin or growth hormone. N. Engl. J. Med. 309: 685.

Kleinman D, Sharon Y, Sarov I, Insler V (1983): Human endometrium: A new method for culturing human endometrium as separate epithelial and stromal components. Arch. Gynecol. 234: 103.

Klijn JGM, Van Geel AN, Sandoz J, De Jong FH (1988): Endocrine, pharmacokinetic and clinical effects of GnRH analogue treatment in patients with malignant and benign breast disease. Gynecological Endocrinology, 2 (Suppl. 1): 49.

Klinefelter HF Jr., Reifenstein EC Jr. , Albright F (1942): Syndrome characterized by gynecomastia, aspermatogenesis without leydigism and increased excretion of follicle stimulating hormone. J. Clin. Endocrinol. Metab. 2: 615.

Kloosterboer HJ, Bergink EW, Muntendam P (1985): A comparative study of the effects of epimestrol and clomiphene on receptor levels in the rat uterus. J.-Sterrid Biochem. 23: 165.

Knobil E (1980): Neuroendocrine control of the menstrual cycle. Recent Prog. Horm. Res. 36: 53.

Knobil E, Plant TM, Wildt L, Belchetz PE, Marshall G (1980): Control of the rhesus monkey menstrual cycle: Permissive role of hypothalamic gonadotropin-releasing hormone. Science 207: 1371.

Koch Y, Barom TC, Chabsieng P, Fridkin M (1974): Biochem. Biophys. Res. Commun. 61: 95.

Koehler RF (1980): Epimestrol in childless marriages. Dtsch. Med. Wschr. 105: 1250–1252.

Kokko E, Janne O, Kauppila A et al. (1981): Cyclic clomiphene citrate treatment lowers cytosol estrogen and progestin receptor concentrations in the endometrium of postmenopausal women on estrogen replacement therapy.

Koppelman MCS, Myles JJ, Kenneet GR et al. (1984): Hyperprolactimemia, amenorrhea and galactorrhea. Am. Intern. Med. 100: 115.

Kraiem Z, Lunenfeld B (1978): Inhibitory action of human follicular fluid on the ovarian accumulation of cyclic AMP. J. Endocrinol. 78: 161–162.

Krause W, Huebner HM, Wichman U (1985): Treatment of oligozoospermia by tamoxiphen: No evidence for direct testicular action. Andrologia, 17: 285.

Kremer J (1968): The in vitro spermatozoal penetration test in fertility investigation. Thesis, University of Groningen.

Kremer J, Jager S, Van Slochteren Draaisma T (1977): Treatment of infertility due to antisperm antibodies. In: V Insler and G Bettendorf (eds), The uterine cervix in reproduction, Thieme Verlag, Stuttgart, p. 249.

Krumme D, Wallner O, Fritz H (1977): Proteinases and proteinase inhibitors in human cervical mucus – selected properties in view of their clinical relevance. In: V Insler and G Bettendorf (eds.), The uterine cervix in reproduction, Georg Thieme Verlag, Stuttgart, pp. 92–100.

Kuhl H, Taubert HD (1975): Inactivation of luteinizing hormone releasing hormone by rat hypothalamic Lcystine arylamidase. Acta Endocrinol. 78: 634.

Kuhl H, Taubert HD (1975a): Short loop feedback mechanism of luteinizing hormone: LH stimulates hypothalamic Lcystine arymidase to inactive LHRH in the rat hypothalamus. Acta Endocrinol. (Copenhagen), 78: 649–663.

Kurachi K, Aono T, Minagawa J et al. (1983): Congenital malformations of newborn infants after clomiphene induced ovulation. Fertil. Steril. 40: 2.

Kvist U (1980): Importance of spermatozoal zinc as temporary inhibitor of sperm nuclear chromatin decondensation ability in man. Acta Physiol. Scand. 109: 79.

Kvist U, Eliasson R (1980): Influence of seminal plasma on chromatin stability of ejaculated human spermatozoa. Int. J. Androl. 3: 130.

L

Lacy D (1972): The endocrine function of the testis, Vol. I. Academic Press, N.Y., London

Lancranjan I (1987): A new approach to initiate the treatment of patients with prolactinomas. In: AR Genazzani, A Volpe and F Facchinetti (eds.), Gynecological Endocrinology, Parthenon Publishing Group, U.K., p. 239.

Landgren BM, Unden AL, Diczfalusy E (1980): Hormonal profile of the cycle in 68 normally menstruating women. Acta Endocrinol. 94: 89.

Landolt AM (1981): Surgical treatment of pituitary prolactinomas: postoperative prolactin and fertility in seventy patients. Fertil. Steril. 35: 620.

Laron Z, Kauli R, Schally AV (1988): Long-term experience with a superactive GnRH analog (DTrp-6-LHRH) in the treatment of precocious puberty - review of 46 patients. Gynecological Endocrinology, 2 (Suppl. 1): 39.

Laschet U, Laschet L, Paarmann HF (1966): Die Gonadotropin- und Steroidhormonaus-scheidung während der Behandlung mit lamethyl 5a andostan 17-ol-3on (mesterolon). Arznei-mittel Forsch. 16: 469.

Laschet U, Laschet L (1968): The effect of mesterolone on gonadotropin and steroid excretion. Proc. 3. Meeting International Study Group Steroid Hormone 3: 169.

Laufer N, Yaffe H, Margalioth EJ, Livshin J, Ben David M, Shenker JG (1981): Effect of bromocryptine treatment on male infertility associated with hyperprolactinemia. Arch. Androl. 6: 343.

LaVecchia C, Franceschi S, Decarli A, Gallus G, Tognoni G (1984): Risk factors for endometrial cancer at different ages. J. Natl. Cancer Inst. 3: 667-671. cp255.

Lee HY (1976): Clinical experience of vaso-vasostomy in Korea. Proc. Internat. Congr. Andrology CIDA, ECO, Barcelona, p. 86.

Lee W, Blandau RJ, Verdugo P (1977): Laser light-scattering studies of cervical mucus. In: V Insler and G Bettendorf (eds.), The uterine cervix in reproduction, Georg Thieme Publishers, Stuttgart, pp. 68-77.

Leethem JH, Rakoff AE (1948): Studies on antihormone specificity with particular reference to gonadotropic therapy in the female. J. Clin. Endocrinol. Metab. 8: 262.

Lemberger L, Crabtree RE (1979): Pharmacological effects in man of a potent, long-acting dopamine receptor agonist. Science, 205: 1151.

Lequin L, Mendels E, Trimbos Kemper G, Naaktgeboren N, Helmerhost F, Van Hall E (1986): Oestrogens in urine or plasma to monitor ovarian response to exogenous gonadotropins (Abstract). Serono Symposium on the control of follicular development, ovarian and luteal function: lessons from in vitro fertilization.

Levalle O, Bokser L, Pacenza N, Aszenmil G, Fiszlejder L, Chervin A, Guitelman A (1984): Restoration and maintenance of spermatogenesis by human chorionic gonadotropin therapy in patients with hypothalamohypophyseal damage. Andrologia 16: 303.

Lewin LM, Beer R (1975): Semiquantitative paper chromatography assay for inositol and fructose: A method for evaluating prostatic and vesicular contributions to human seminal fluid. Isr. J. Med. Sci. 11: 523.

Lewis-Jones DI, Lynch RV, Machin DC, Desmond AD (1987): Improvement in semen quality in infertile males after treatment with tamoxifen. Andrologia 19: 86.

Lewis UJ, Singh RNP, Sinha YN et al. (1971): Electrophoretic evidence for human prolactin. J. Clin. Endocrinol. 32: 153.

Leyendecker G, Struve T, Plotz EJ (1980): Induction of ovulation with chronic intermittent (pulsatile) administration of LHRH in women with hypothalamic and hyperprolactinemic amenorrhea. Arch. Gynecol. 229: 177.

Leyendecker G, Wildt L, Hansmann M (1980b): Pregnancies following chronic intermittent (pulsatile) administration of GnRH by means of a portable pump - a new approach to the treatment of infertility in hypothalamic amenorrhea. J. Clin. Endocrinol. Metab. 51: 1214.

Lin T, Calkins JK, Morris PL, Vale W, Bardin CW (1989): Regulation of Leydig cell function in primary culture by inhibin and activin. Endocrinology 125: 2134.

Lin T, Haskell J, Vinson N, Terracio I (1986): Direct stimulatory effects of insulin-like growth factor-I on Leydig cell steroidogenesis in primary culture. Biochem. Biophys. Res. Commun. 137: 950.

Ling N, Ying SY, Ueno N, Shimasaki S, Esch F, Hotta M, Guillemin R (1986): Pituitary FSH is released by a heterodimer of the beta subunits from two forms of inhibin. Nature 321, 779.

Lipsett MB (1971): Steroid secretion by the gonads in man. In: VHT James and L Martini (eds.): Hormonal steroids, Excerpta. Med. Found. Intern. Congr. Ser. 219.

Liu TC, Jackson GL (1978): Modification of luteinizing hormone biosynthesis by gonadotropin releasing hormone, cycloheximide and actinomycin D. Endocrinology 103: 1253.

Lloyd HM, Meares JD, Jacobi J (1975): Effects of estrogen and bromocriptine on in vivo secretion and mitosis in prolactin cells. Nature 255: 497.

Lopata A, Gronow MJ, Johnston WIH, McBain JC, Speirs AL, Leung PS (1986): In vitro fertilization and embryo implantation. In: V Insler and B Lunenfeld (eds.), Infertility: male and female, Churchill Livingstone, London, p. 496.

Lopez JRC, Silva LG, Iglesias JR, Lobo CN, Alves Neto J (1981): Clinical trial with epimestrol. J. Bras. Ginecol. 91: 71-74.

Louis BG, Griswold MD, Fritz B (1975): 57th Annual Meeting. Endocrine Society, p. A-177.

Louvet JP, Harman SM, Schreiber JR, Ross GT (1975): Evidence for a role of androgens in follicular maturation. Endocrinology 97: 366.

Louvet JP, Vaitukaitis JL (1975): Induction of follicle stimulating hormone (FSH) receptors in rat ovaries by estrogen priming. Abstracts of the 57th Annual Meeting of the Endocrine Society, New York, p. 135.

Ludvik W (1976): Andrologie. Thieme Verlag, Stuttgart.

Ludwig G, Weigl H, Nuri M, Peters HJ (1974): Vergleichende Bestimmung der Spermaplasma Fruktose nach der enzymatischen und der dünnschichtchromatographischen Methode. Urologie 13: 177.

Lunenfeld B (1963): Treatment of anovulation by human gonadotropins. Int. J. Gynecol. Obstet. 1: 153.

Lunenfeld B, Eshkol A (1967): Immunology of human chorionic gonadotropin (hCG). Vitamins and Hormones 25: 137–190.

Lunenfeld B, Insler V, Rabau E (1970): Die Prinzipien der Gonadotropintherapie. Acta Endocrinol. Suppl. 148: 52–101.

Lunenfeld B, Weissenberg R (1972): The use of gonadotropins in the induction of spermatogenesis. In: FIG Prunty, H Gordina Hill (eds.), Modern trends in endocrinology, London, Butterworths.

Lunenfeld B, Insler V, Eshkol A, Birenboim N (1974): Pituitary responsiveness to gonadotropin releasing hormone. Hormone and Metabolic Research, Supplementum 5: 184.

Lunenfeld B, Glezerman M (1977): Versuch eines algorithmischen Ansatzes zur Diagnose männlicher Fertilitätsstörungen. Akta Dermatol. 3: 119.

Lunenfeld B, Insler V (1978): Diagnosis and treatment of functional infertility, Grosse Verlag, Berlin.

Lunenfeld B, Glezerman M (1981): Diagnose und Therapie männlicher Fertilitätsstörungen. Grosse Verlag, Berlin.

Lunenfeld B, Serr DM, Mashiah S, Oelsner G, Blankstein J, Dor J, Frenkel Y, Ben-Raphael Z, Tikotzky D, Snyder M (1981): Therapy with gonadotropins: Where are we today. In: V Insler and G Bettendorf (eds.), Advances in diagnosis and treatment of infertility, Elsevier, North Holland, New York, p. 27.

Lunenfeld B, Eshkol A, Glezerman M (1982): Male climacteric. In: K Brandhauer, J Frick (eds.), Handbook of Urology, Disturbances of Male fertility, XVIth ed., Springer Verlag, Berlin, Heidelberg, New York, p. 421.

Lunenfeld B, Mashiah S, Blankstein J (1985): Induction of ovulation with gonadotropins. In: R Shearman (eds.), Clinical Reproductive Endocrinology, Churchill Livingstone, p. 523.

Lunenfeld B, Blankstein J, Shadmi A (1986): FSH biosynthesis and physiology. Actualites Gynecologis, 16: 7.

Lunenfeld B, Blankstein J, Ron E et al. (1987): Short and long term survey of patients treated with HMG/HCG and follow up of offspring. In: AR Genazziani, A Volpe and F Facchinetti (eds.), Proceedings of the First International Congress on Gynecological Endocrinology, p. 459.

Lunenfeld E and Lunenfeld B (1988): Modern approaches to the diagnosis and management of anovulation. Int. J. Fert. 33: 308–318.

Lunenfeld B (1990): Past present and future of gonadotrophins. In: Mashiah S, Ben-Rafael Z, Laufer N, Schenker JG (eds.), Advances in Assisted Reproductive Technologies. Plenum Press, New York, p. 39–44.

Lunenfeld B, Glezerman M (1992): Diagnosis of male infertility. In: V Insler and B Lunenfeld (eds): Infertility – male and female, Churchill Livingstone, Edinburgh – London – Melbourne – New York (in press)

Lytton B, Mroueh A (1966): Treatment of oligospermia with urinary gonadotropin – a preliminary report. Fertil. Steril. 17: 696.

Lytton B, Kase N (1966): Effects of human menopausal gonadotropin on a eunuchoidal male. Eng. J. Med. 274: 1061.

M

Macdonald RR (1969): Cyclic changes in cervical mucus. J. Obstet. Gynaecol. Brit. Cwlth. 76: 1090–1099.

MacGregor AH, Johnson JE, Bunde CA (1968): Further clinical experience with clomiphene citrate. Fertil. Steril. 19: 616.

MacLeod J (1965): The semen examination. Clin. Obstet. Gynecol. 8: 115.

MacLeod J, Gold RZ (1951): Semen quality in 1000 men of known fertility and 800 cases of infertile marriage. Fertil. Steril. 2: 115.

MacLeod J (1969): Further observations on the role of varicocele in human male infertility. Fertil. Steril. 20: 545.

MacLeod J (1979): The effect of urinary gonadotrophins following hypophysectomy and hypogonadotrophic eunuchoidism. In: E Romberg and CA Paulsen (eds.), The Human Testis. Plenum Press, New York.

MacLeod J, Pazianos A, Ray BS (1964): Restoration of human spermatogenesis by menopausal gonadotrophins. Lancet 1: 1197.

MacLeod J, Pazianos A, Ray B (1966): Restoration of human spermatogenesis and of the reproductive tract with urinary gonadotrophins following hypophysectomy. Fertil. Steril. 17: 7

MacLeod RM, Fontham EH, Lehmeyer JE (1970): Prolactin and growth hormone production as influenced by catecholamines and agents that affect brain catecholamines. Neuroendocrinology 6: 283.

MacLeod SC, Mitton DM, Parker AS, Tupper WRC (1970): Experience with induction of ovulation. Am. J. Obstet. Gynecol. 108: 814–824.

Macomber D, Sander MR (1929): The spermatozoa count. N. Eng. J. Med. 200: 981.

Maia H Jr., Maia H, Barbossa IC, Coutinho EM, Almeida P (1983): Induction of ovulation with epimestrol and clomiphene in patients resistant to clomiphene alone. In: RF Harrison (ed.), Abstracts of 11th World Congress on Fertility and Sterility, Dublin, June/July, 1983, Abstr. No. 516.

Maisey NM, Bingham J, Marks V, English J, Chakroborty J (1981): Clinical efficacy of testosterone undecanoate in male hypogonadism. Clin. Endocrinol. (Oxf.) 14: 625.

Major P, Kilpatrick R (1972): Review – cyclic AMP and hormone action. J. Endocr. 52: 593.

Makler A (1978): A new multiple exposure photography method for sperm motility determination. Fertil. Steril. 30: 192.

Makler A (1978a): A new chamber for rapid sperm count and motility estimation. Fertil. Steril. 30: 313.

Makler A (1978b): The thickness of microscopically examined seminal sample and its relationship to sperm motility examination. Int. J. Androl. 1: 213.

Makler A, Glezerman M, Lunenfeld B (1977): The fertile eunuch syndrome – an isolated Leydig cell failure? Andrologia 9: 163.

Makler A, Tatcher M, Mohiliver J (1980): Sperm semiautoanalyses by combination of the MEP and computer techniques. Int. J. Fertil. 25: 62.

Mann EC, McLarn WD, Hayt DB (1961): The physiology and clinical significance of the uterine isthmus. Am. J. Obstet. Gynecol. 81: 209–222.

Mann T (1964): The Biochemistry of Semen and of the Male Reproductive Tract. Methuen, London.

Mann T (1973): Energy requirement of spermatozoa and the cervical environment. In: RJ Blandau and K Moghissi (eds.), The biology of the cervix, The University of Chicago Press, Chicago and London, pp. 329–338.

Mann T, Lutvak-Mann C (1981): Male reproductive function and semen. Springer Verlag, Berlin, Heidelberg, New York.

March CM, Tredway DR, Mishell DR (1976): Effect of clomiphene citrate upon amount and duration of human menopausal gonadotropin therapy. Am. J. Obstet. Gynecol. 125: 699.

March CM, Kletzky OA, Davajan V et al. (1981): Longitudinal evaluation of patients with untreated prolactin secreting pituitary adenomas. Am. J. Obstet. Gynecol. 139: 835.

Marcus CC, Marcus SL (1965): The cervical factor in infertility. Clin. Obstet. Gynecol. 8: 15–31.

Marcus CC, Marcus SL (1968): The cervical factor. In: SJ Behrman and RW Kistner (eds), Progress in fertility, Little, Brown & Co. Boston, pp. 21–62.

Margalioth E, Laufer N, Persistz E, Gaulayev B, Shemesh A, Schenker JG (1983): Treatment of oligoasthenospermia with human chorionic gonadotropin; Hormonal profiles and results. Fertil. Steril. 39: 841.

Marshall JR, Jacobson A (1970): A technique of dose selection in ovulation induction with HMG. In: JK Butler (ed.), Developments in pharmacological and clinical uses of human gonadotrophins, GD Searle & Co., High Wycombe, England, pp. 141–148.

Marshall GR, Nieschlag E (1987): The role of FSH in male reproduction. In: AR Sheth (ed.), Inhibins: Isolation, estimation and physiology, Vol I. CRC Press, Boca Raton, p. 3.

Martini L, Massa R, Motta M, Zanisi M (1974): Male fertility and sterility. Academic Press, London, New York, San Francisco.

Mashiter K, Adams E, Beard M et al. (1977): Bromocriptine inhibits prolactin and growth hormone release by human pituitary tumors in culture. Lancet 2: 197.

Masson PL (1973): Carbohydrate component of cervical mucus. In: M Elstein, KS Moghissi and R Borth (eds.), Cervical mucus in human reproduction, Scriptor, Copenhagen, pp. 82–92.

Masters WH, Johnson VE (1966): Human sexual response. Little, Brown & Co., Boston.

Matsumoto S (1962): Evaluation of clinical and laboratory tests for menstrual disorders. The Gunma Journal of Medical Sciences 11: 95–149.

Matsuo H, Baba Y, Nair RMG, Arimura A, Schally AV (1971a): Structure of the porcine LH and FSH releasing factor: I. The proposed amino acid sequence. Biochem. Biophys. Res. Commun. 43: 1334.

Matsuo H, Arimura A, Nair RMG, Schally AV (1971b): Synthesis of the porcine LH and FSH releasing hormone by the solid phase method. Biochem. Biophys. Res. Commun. 45: 828.

Matthews CD, Broom TJ, Crawshaw KM, Hopkins RE, Kerin JFP, Svigos JM (1979): The influence of insemination timing and semen characteristics on the efficiency of a donor insemination program. Fertil. Steril. 31: 45.

Mattner PE (1968): The distribution of spermatozoa and leucocytes in the female genital tract in goats and cattle. J. Reprod. Fertil. 17: 253.

Mauss J (1974): Ergebnisse der Behandlung von Fertilitätsstörungen des Mannes mit Mesterolon oder einem Placebo. Arzneim. Forsch. 24: 1338.

Max D, Seely J, Swanson L, Brauneller R (1988): Clinical studies of leuprolide depot formulation in metastatic prostatic cancer. Gynecological Endocrinology, 2 (Suppl. 1): 80.

McGuire WL, De la Garcia M (1973): Similarity of the estrogen receptor in human and rat mammary carcinoma. J. Clin. Endocrinol. Metab. 36: 548.

McKeown J (1960): Malformations in a population observed for five years. In: Foundations Symposium on Congenital Malformations. J. & A. Churchill Ltd., London, p. 2.

McLachlan RI, Matsumoto AM, Burger HG, De Kretser DM, Bremner WJ (1988): Relative roles of follicle stimulating hormone and luteinizing hormone in the control of inhibin secretion in normal men. J. Clin. Invest. 82: 880.

McNatty KP, McNeilly AS, Sawyers RS (1977): Prolactin and progesterone secretion by human granulosa cells in vitro. In: PG Crosignani, C Robyn (eds.), Prolactin and Human Reproduction. Serono Symposia Proceedings, London, Academic Press, Vol. 11.

Mehan DJ, Chehval MJ (1982): Human chorionic gonadotropin in the treatment of the infertile man. J. Urol. 128: 60.

Mehta AE, Tolis G (1979): Pharmacology of bromocriptine in health and disease. Drugs 17: 313.

Meldrum DR, Chang RJ, Lu J, Vale W, Rivier J, Judd HL (1982): Medical oophorectomy using a long-acting GnRH agonist – a possible new approach to treatment of endometriosis. J. Clin. Endocrinol. Metab. 54: 1081.

Menard RH, Loriaux DL, Bartter FC, Gillette JR (1978): The effect of administration of spironolactone on the concentration of plasma testosterone, estradiol and cortisone in male dogs. Steroid 31: 771.

Mettler L, Schirvani D (1975): Macrophage migration inhibitory factor in female sterility. Am. J. Obstet. Gynecol. 121: 117–120.

Michelson L, Roland S, Koets P (1955): The effect of cortisone on the infertile male. Fertil. Steril. 6: 493.

Micic S, Dotlic R (1985): Evaluation of sperm parameters in clinical trial with clomiphene citrate of oligospermic men. J. Urol. 133: 221.

Mickelson TJ, Baustian CL, Cameron WJ (1984): Preliminary report of the disposition of clomiphene in healthy human subjects. Fertil. Steril. 41: 935.

Mickelson TJ, Kroboth PD, Cameron WJ, Dittert LW, Chungi V, Manberg PJ (1986): Single dose pharmacokinetics of clomiphene citrate in normal volunteers. Fertil. Steril. 46: 392.

Mies R, Krempl S (1980): Die Wirkung von Testosterone Undecanoat beim männlichen Hypogonadismus. Med. Welt 31: 619.

Miller D, Reid RR, Cetel NS et al. (1983): Conception following ovulation by pulsatile administration of low doses of gonadotropin releasing hormone in women with hypothalamic amenorrhea. J.A.M.A.

Moghissi KS, Neuhaus OW (1966): Cyclic changes of cervical mucus proteins. Am. J. Obstet. Gynecol. 96: 91–95.

Moghissi KS (1973): Sperm migration through the human cervix. In: M Elstein, KS Moghissi and R Borth (eds.), Cervical mucus in human reproduction, Scriptor, Copenhagen, pp. 128–152.

Mogulesvky JA, Enero MA, Szwarcfarm B, Dosoretz D (1974): Effects of castration and testosterone in vitro on the hypothalamic synthesis of different peptide fractions. J. Endocrin. 64: 1.

Moodbidri SB, Vijayalakshmi S, Bandivdekar AH, Sheth AR (1981): Inhibition of hypothalamic GnRH sythesis by inhibin. Experientia 37: 525.

Moodbidri SB, Bandivdekar AH, Sheth AR (1987): Isolation and characterisation of Inhibins: Progress and problems. In: Sheth AR (ed.), Inhibins: Isolation, estimation and physiology, Vol I. CRC Press, Boca Raton, p. 27.

Morris DW, Abdulwahid NA, Jacobs HS (1985): Human chorionic gonadotropin support of spermatogenesis following pulsatile LHRH therapy. J. Endocrinol. 104 (Suppl.): 21.

Mortimer D, Templeton AA, Lenton EA, Coleman RA (1982): Influence of abstinence and ejaculation to analysis delay on semen analysis: parameters of suspected infertile men. Arch. of Androl. 8: 251.

Moudgal NR, Moyle WR, Greep RO (1971): Specific binding of LH to Leydig tumor cells. Biol. Chem. 246: 4983.

Moult PJA, Rees LH, Besser GM (1982): Pulsatile gonadotrophin secretion in hyperprolactinemic amenorrhea and the response to bromocriptine therapy. Clin. Endocrinol. 16: 153.

Moyle WR, Moudgal NR, Greep RO (1971): Cessation of steroidogenesis in Leydig cell tumors after removal of LH and adenosine cyclic 3'5'-monophosphate.

Mozes M, Bogakowsky H, Antevi E, Lunenfeld B, Rabau E, Serr DM, David A, Salomy M (1965): Thromboembolic phenomena after ovarian stimulation with human gonadotrophins. Lancet 2: 1213–1215.

Mroueh A, Siller-Khodr TM (1977): Bromocriptine therapy in cases of amenorrhea galactorrhea. Am. J. Obstet. Gynec. 127: 291–298.

Murphy DP, Torrano EF (1966): Donor insemination. A study of 112 women. Fertil. Steril. 17: 273.

Murray M, Osmond-Clarke F (1971): Pregnancy results following treatment with clomiphene citrate. J. Obstet. Gynaecol. Brit. Cwlth. 78: 1108–1114.

N

Naftolin F, Ryan KJ, Petro Z (1972): Aromatization of androstendione by the anterior hypothalamus of adult male and female rats. Endocrinology 90: 295.

Nakhla AM, Mather JP, Janne OA, Bardin CW (1984): Estrogen and androgen receptors in Sertoli, Leydig, myoid and epithelial cells: effects of time in culture and cell density. Endocrinology 115: 121.

Naor Z, Childs GV, Leifer AM et al. (1982): Gonadotropin releasing hormone binding and activation of enriched population of pituitary gonadotrophs. Mol. Cell. Endocrinol. 25: 85.

Nappi C, Mercorio F, Trezza G (1981): Cervical mucus during ovulatory treatment with epimestrol. J. Steroid. Biochem. 14, No. 11, p. XXVIII, Abstr. 55.

Navot D, Schenker JG (1985): The role of in vitro fertilization in unexplained and immunological infertility. Contrib. Gynecol. Obstet. 14: 160-169.

Navot D, Margalioth EJ, Laufer N, Birkenfeld A, Relou A, Rosler A, Shenker JG (1987): Direct correlation between plasma renin activity and severity of the ovarian hyperstimulation syndrome. Fertil. Steril. 48 (1): 57-61.

Neale C, Bettendorf G, Trou G (1970): Clinical studies on bis-(P ace toxyphenyl)cyclohexylidmethane (sexovid) and on 6-chloro-9 beta,6-10αpregna-1,4,6-triene-3,20-dione (Ro 4-8347). Bull. Schweiz. Akad. Med. Wiss. 25: 545.

Negro-Vilar A (1980): Prolactin and the growth of prostate and seminal vesicles. In: E Spring-Mills, ESE Hafez (eds.), Human reproductive medicine. Male accessory glands. Elsevier, North Holland Biomedical Press, Amsterdam, p. 223.

Nichols JB (1952): Statistics of births in the USA, 1915 - 1948. Am. J. Obstet. Gynecol. 64: 376.

Nicosia SV (1981): An in vivo and in vitro structural functional analysis of cervical mucus secretion. Reproduccion 5: 261-280.

Nie NH, Maldi Hull C, Jenkins JG, Steinberger K, Bent DH (1975): Statistical Package for the Social Sciences, Ch. 23. McGrawHill Co., New York.

Nieschlag E, Freischem CW (1982): Androgen therapy in hypogonadism and infertility. In: J Bain, WB Schill, L Schwarzstein (eds.), Treatment of male infertility. Springer Verlag, Berlin - Heidelberg - New York, p. 103.

Nikkanen V, Groenroos M, Suominen J, Multamäki S (1979): Silent infection in male accesssory genital organs and male infertility. Andrologia 11: 236.

Nillius SJ, Wide L (1979): Effects of prolonged luteinizing hormone releasing hormone therapy on follicular maturation, ovulation and corpus luteum function in amenorrhoeic women with anorexia nervosa. Upsalla J. Med. Sci. 84: 21.

Nillius SJ, Skarin G, Wide L (1981): Gonadotropin Releasing Hormone and its Agonists for Induction of Follicular Maturation and Ovulation. In: V Insler and G Bettendorf (eds), Advances in Diagnosis and Treatment of Infertility. Elsevier, North Holland, New York, p. 5.

Nitschke-Dabelstein S, Sturm G, Prinz H, Buchholz R (1981): Plasma 17-beta estradiol and plasma progesterone as indicators of cyclic changes in the follicle bearing ovary during the periovulatory phase. In: V Insler, G Bettendorf, KH Geissler (eds.), Advances in diagnosis and treatment of infertility, Elsevier, North Holland, New York, pp. 57-64.

Noyes RW (1966): Endometrial dating for the detection of ovulation. In: RB Greenblatt (ed.), Ovulation, Lippincott, Philadelphia, p. 319.

Nyboe Andersen A, Schioler V, Hertz J et al. (1982): Effect of metoclopramide induced hyperprolactinemia on the gonadotrophic response to estradiol and LRH. Acta Endocrinol. (Copenhagen). 100: 1.

O

Odeblad E (1966): MicroNMR in high permanent magnetic fields. Acta Obstet. Gynecol. Scand. 45 (Suppl. 2): 127-160.

Odeblad E (1973): Biophysical techniques of assessing cervical mucus and microstructure of cervical epithelium. In: M Elstein, KS Moghissi and R Borth (eds.), Cervical mucus in human reproduction, Scriptor, Copenhagen, pp. 58-74.

O'Herlihy C, Pepperell RJ, Brown JB, Smith MA, Sandri L, McBain JC (1981): Incremental clomiphene therapy: a new method for treating persistent anovulation. Obstet. Gynecol. 58: 535.

O'Herlihy C, Pepperell RJ, Robinson M (1982): Ultrasound timing of HCG administration in clomiphene stimulated cycles. Obstet. Gynecol. 59: 40.

Okuyama A, Namiki M, Koide T, Itatani H, Mizutani S, Sonoda T, Aono I, Matsumoto K (1981): A simple hCG stimulation test for normal and hypogonadal males. Arch. Androl. 6: 75.

Oosterlinck W, Wallijn, Wyndale JJ (1976): The concentration of doxycycline in human prostate gland and its importance in the treatment of prostatis. I. Intern. Congress of Andrology, Barcelona (Abstract).

Orth J, Christensen AK (1978): Autoradiographic localisation of specifically bound 125-I labeled follicle stimulating hormone on spermatogonia of the rat testes. Endocrinology 103: 1944.

P

Pardo M, Barri PN, Bancells N, Coroleu B, Buxadras C, Pomerol JM Jr, Sabater J (1988): Spermatozoa selection in discontinuous percoll gradients for use in artificial insemination. Fertil. Steril. 49: 505.

Parmar H, Edwards L, Phillips RH, Allen L, Lightman S (1988): Orchidectomy versus long acting DTrp-6-LHRH in advanced prostatic cancer. Gynecological Endocrinology, 2 (Suppl. 1): 56.

Patanelli DJ (ed.) (1978): Proceedings of hormonal control of male fertility. DHEW publication No. 78-1097, National Institutes of Health, Bethesda.

Paulsen CA (1980): In: MA Belsey, R Eliasson, AJ Gallegos, KS Moghissi, CA Paulsen,

MRN Prasad (eds.), Laboratory Manual for the Examination of Human Semen and Semen-Cervical Mucus Interaction, Press Concern, Singapore, p. 8.

Paulson JD, Polakoski KL, Leto S (1979): Further characterisation of glass wool column filtration of human semen. Fertil. Steril. 32, 125.

Paz G, Kogosowski A, Yogev L, Homonnai ZT (1986): The use of laboratory techniques in improvement of sperm quality. In: JD Paulson, A Negro-Vilar, E Lucena, L Martini (eds.): Andrology – Male Fertility and Sterility. Academic Press, Orlando – San Diego – New York – Austin – Boston – London – Sydney – Tokyo – Toronto, p. 377.

Pearson KC (1981): Mental disorders from low dose bromocriptine. N. Engl. J. Med. 305: 173.

Pepperell RJ, Evans JH, Brown JB, Bright MI, Smith M, Burger HG, Healy D (1977): A study of the effects of bromocriptine on serum prolactin, follicle stimulating hormone and luteinizing hormone and on ovarian responsiveness to exogenous gonadotropins in anovulatory women. Br. J. Obstet. Gynaecol. 84: 456.

Perkes J (1977): Bromocriptine. In: N Harper, A Simmond (eds.), Recent Advances in Drug Research, Academic Press, New York, p. 247.

Perry GM, Glezerman M, Insler V (1977): Selective filtration of abdominal spermatozoa by the cervical mucus in vitro. In: V Insler and G Bettendorf (eds.), The uterine cervix in reproduction, Georg Thieme Verlag, Stuttgart, pp. 118-128.

Perryman RL, Thorner MO (1981): The effects of hyperprolactinemia on sexual and reproductive function in men. J. Androl. 3: 233.

Person BH (1965): Clinical effects of bis-(pacetoxyphenyl) cyclohexylidenemethane (Compound F 6066) on hormone excretion in postmenopausal women. Acta Soc. Med. Upsalien 70: 1.

Phillips LL, Gladstone W, Vande Wiele R (1975): Studies on the regulation and fibrinolytic systems in hyperstimulation syndrome after administration of human gonadotropins. J. Reprod. Med. 14: 138-143.

Pigman W, Moschera J (1973): The nature and functions of the epithelial mucus glycoproteins. In: RJ Blandau and K Moghissi (eds.), The biology of cervix, The University of Chicago Press, Chicago and London, pp. 143-172.

Pildes RB (1965): Induction of ovulation with clomiphene. Am. J. Obstet. Gynecol. 91: 466-479.

Pimstone B, Epstein S, Hamilton SM et al. (1977): Metabolic clearance and plasma half disappearance time of exogenous gonadotropin releasing hormone in normal subjects and in patients with liver disease and chronic renal failure. J. Clin. Endocrinol. Metab. 44: 356.

Pohl CR, Richardson DW, Hutchinson JS et al. (1983): Hypophysiotropic signal frequency and the functioning of the pituitary ovarian system in the rhesus monkey. Endocrinology 112: 2076.

Polakoski KL, Zaneveld LJD (1977): Biochemical examination of the human ejaculate. In: ESE Hafez (ed.), Techniques of Human Andrology. Elsevier, North Holland Biomed Press, Amsterdam, p. 265.

Polatti F (1981): Bromocriptin and epimestrol in MAP negative secondary amenorrheas. Clin. Exp. Obstet. Gynecol. 8: 164-166.

Polishuk WZ, Schenker JG (1969): Ovarian overstimulation syndrome. Fertil. Steril. 20: 443.

Poon WW, McCoshen RV (1985): Variances in mucus architecture as a cause of cervical factor infertility. Fertil. Steril. 44: 361.

Potashnik G, Glassner M, Holzberg G, Insler V (1986): Personal communication of unpublished data.

Potashnik G, Yanai-Inber I (1987): Dibromochloropropane (DBCP): An eight year reevaluation of testicular function and reproductive performance. Fertil. Steril. 47: 317.

Potts I (1957): The mechanism of retrograde ejaculation. Med. J. Aust. 1: 495.

Pryor JP (1981): Semen analysis. Clin. Obstet. Gynecol. 8: 571.

Pusch HH, Puerstner P, Haas J (1986a): Treatment of asthenospermia with human chorionic gonadotropin. Andrologia 18: 201.

Pusch HH, Haas J, Puerstner P (1986b): Results of treatment of oligozoospermia with clomiphene citrate. Andrologia 18: 561.

Pusch HH (1989): Oral Treatment of Oligozoospermia with Testosterone Undecanoate: Results of a Double Blind Placebo Controlled Trial. Andrologia 21: 76.

Q

Quigley MM (1985): Selection of agents for enhanced follicular recruitment in an in vitro fertilization and embryo replacement treatment program. Ann. N.Y. Acad. Sci. 442: 96.

Quinlivan WLG, Preciado K, Lorraine Long T, Sullivan H (1982): Separation of human X- and Y-spematozoa by albumin gradients and sephadex chromatography. Fertil. Steril. 37: 104.

R

Rabau E, Serr DM, Mashiach S et al. (1967): Current concepts in the treatment of anovulation. Br. Med. J. Clin. Res. 4: 446-449.

Rabau E, Lunenfeld B, Insler V (1971): The treatment of fertility disturbances with special reference to the use of human gonadotropins. In: ChA Joel (ed.), Fertility disturbances in men and women, Karger, Basel, pp. 508-540.

Racagni G, Apud JA, Locatelli V et al. (1979): GABA of CNS origin in the rat anterior pituitary inhibits prolactin secretion. Nature 281: 575.

Ramasharma K, Sairam MR, Seidah NH, Chretien M, Manjunath P, Schiller PW, Yamshiro D, Li CH (1984): Isolation, structure and synthesis of a human seminal plasma peptide with inhibin-like activity. Science 223: 1199.

Raymond V, Beaulieu M, Labrie F et al. (1978): Potent antidopaminergic activity of estradiol at the pituitary level on prolactin release. Science 200: 1173.

Rehan NE, Sobrero AJ, Fertig JW (1975): The semen of fertile men: Statistical analysis of 1300 men. Fertil. Steril. 26: 492.

Reichman J, Insler V, Serr DM (1973a): A modified in vitro spermatozoal penetration test; 2. Application in fertility investigations. Int. J. Fertil. 18: 241-245.

Reichman J, Insler V, Serr DM (1973b): A modified in vitro spermatozoal penetration test. Int. J. Fertil. 18: 232-240.

Retieff PJM (1950): Physiology of micturition and ejaculation. S. Afr. Med. J. 24: 509.

Richards JS, Midgley AR (1976): Protein hormone action: a key to understanding ovarian follicular and luteal cell development. Biol. Reprod. 14: 82-94.

Richter M, Haning RV Jr., Shapiro SS (1984): Artificial donor insemination: fresh versus frozen semen; the patient as her own control. Fertil. Steril. 41: 277.

Rieser C (1961): The etiology of retrograde ejaculation and a method for insemination. Fertil. Steril. 12: 488.

Risbridger GP, Clements J, Robertson DM, Drummond AE, Muir J, Burger HG, De Kretser DM (1989): Immuno and bioactive inhibin alpha subunit expression in rat Leydig cell cultures. Moll. Cell. Endocrinol. 66: 119.

Ritchie WGM (1985): Ultrasound in the evaluation of normal and induced ovulation. Fertil. Steril. 43: 167.

Rivier J, McClintock R, Vaughan J, Yamamoto G, Anderson H, Spiess J, Vale W, Voglmayr J, Cheng CY, Bardin CW (1986): Partial purification of Inhibin from ovine rete testis fluid. In: GL Zatuchni, A Goldsmith, JM Spieler, JJ Sciarra (eds.), Male contraception: Advances and future aspects. Harper and Row, Philadelphia, p. 401.

Roberts V, Meunier H, Sawchenko PE, Vale W (1989): Differential production and regulation of inhibin subunits in rat testicular cell types. Endocrinology 125: 2350.

Robertson JFR, Blamey RW (1988): GnRH analogues in breast cancer. Gynecological Endocrinology, 2 (Suppl. 1): 50.

Robertson S, Birrel W, Grant A (1977): Fewer multiple pregnancies using clomiphene/human gonadotropin sequence. Fertil. Steril. (Abstr.), 28: 294.

Robson IM, Schonberg A (1937): Oestrons reactions, including mating, produced by triphenyl ethylene. Nature 140: 196.

Roennberg L (1980): The effect of clomiphen citrate on different sperm parameters and serum hormone levels in preselected infertile men: a controlled double blind crossover study. Int. J. Androl. 3: 479.

Ron E, Lunenfeld B, Menczer J, Serr D, Katz L (1985): Cancer incidence in a cohort of infertile women. Am. J. Epidemiol. 2: 516.

Rondell P (1974): Role of steroid synthesis in the process of ovulation. Biol. Reprod. 10: 199-215.

Rosemberg E (1976): Gonadotropin therapy in male infertility. In: ESE Hafez (ed.), Human semen and fertility regulation in man. Mosby Co., St. Louis, p. 464.

Ross GT, Cargille CM, Lipset MB, Rayford PL, Marshall JR, Strott CA, Rodbard D (1970): Pituitary and gonadal hormones in women during spontaneous and induced ovulatory cycles. Recent Progress in Hormone Research 26: 1-62.

Rowley MJ, Teshima F, Heller CG (1970): Duration of transit of spermatozoa through the human male ductular system. Fertil. Steril. 21: 390.

Ruberg M, Rotsztein WH, Arancibia S et al. (1978): Stimulation of prolactin release by vasoactive intestinal peptide (VIP). Eur. J. Pharmacol. 51: 319.

Rust LA, Israel R, Mishell DR (1974): An individualized graduated therapeutic regimen for clomiphene citrate. Am. J. Obstet. Gynecol. 120: 785-790.

S

Sagle MA, Hamilton-Fairley D, Kiddy DS, Franks S (1991): A comparative, randomized study on low-dose human menopausal gonadotropin and follicle-stimulating hormone in women with polycystic ovarian syndrome. Fertil. Steril. 55: 56-60.

Sanborn BM, Steinberger A, Meistrich WL, Steinberger E (1975): Androgen binding sites in testis fractions as measured by a nuclear exchange assay. J. Ster. Biochem. 6: 1459.

Santamauro AG, Sclavra JJ, Varna AO (1972): A clinical investigation of the semen analysis and postcoital test in the evaluation of male infertility. Fertil. Steril. 23: 245.

Santen RJ (1975): Is aromatization of testosterone to estradiol required for the inhibition of luteinizing hormone secretion in man? J. Clin. Invest. 56: 1555.

Santen RJ, Bardin CW (1973): Episodic luteinizing hormone secretion in man. Pulse analysis, clinical interpretation, physiologic mechanisms. J. Clin. Invest. 52: 2617.

Santiemma V, Casasanta N, Rosati P, Moscardelli S, Iapadre G, Fabbrini A (1984): Response to FSH of human Sertoli cells in culture. In: W Thompson, RF Harrison, J Bonnar (eds.), The male factor in human infertility, MTP Press Ltd, Lancaster – Boston – The Hague – Dordrecht, p. 85.

Sasson S, Notides CA (1982): The inhibition of the estrogen receptors positive cooperative (3H) estradiol binding by the antagonist clomiphene. J. Biol. Chem. Vol. 25, 19: 11540.

Sato T, Ibuki Y, Hirono M, Igarashi M, Matsumoto S (1969): Induction of ovulation with Sexorid (compound F. 6066) and its mode of action. Fertil. Steril. 20: 965.

Sauer MW, Zeffer KB, Buster JH, Sokol RZ (1988): Effect of abstinence on sperm motility in normal men. Am. J. Obstet. Gynecol. 158: 604.

Sayfan J, Halevy A, Oland J, Nathan H (1984): Varicocele and left renal vein compression. Fertil. Steril. 41: 411.

Scammel GE, Stendronska J, Dempsey A (1982): Successful pregnancies using human serum albumin following retrograde ejaculation. Fertil. Steril. 37: 277.

Schally AV, Arimura A, Baba Y, Nair RMG, Matsuo H, Redding TW, Debeljuk L (1971a): Isolation and properties of the LH releasing hormone. Biochem. Biophys. Res. Commu. 43: 393–399.

Schally AV, Baba Y, Redding TW (1971b): Studies on the enzymatic and chemical inactivation of hypothalamic follicle stimulating hormone releasing hormone. Neuroendocr. 8: 70.

Schally AV, Arimura A, Kastin AJ, Matsuo H, Redding T, Nair RMG, Debeljuk L, White WF (1971c): Gonadotropin releasing hormone: One polypeptide regulates secretion of luteinizing and follicle stimulating hormones. Science 173: 1036.

Schally AV, Coy DH, Meyers CA (1978): Hyptohalamic regulatory hormones. Ann. Rev. Biochem. 47: 89–128.

Scharf M, Graff G, Kuzminski T (1971): Quinestrol therapy in hypomucorrhea due to clomiphene. Am. J. Obstet. Gynecol. 110: 423.

Schellen AM (1982): Clomiphen citrate in the treatment of male infertility. In: J Bain, WB Schill, L Schwarzstein (eds.), Treatment of male infertility. Springer Verlag, Berlin – Heidelberg – New York, p. 33.

Schellen TCM (1970): Results with mesterolone in the treatment of disturbances of spermatogenesis. Andrologia 2: 1.

Schenken RS, Hodgen GD (1983): Follicle stimulating hormone induced ovarian hyperstimulation in monkeys: blockade of the luteinizing hormone surge. J. Clin. Endocrinol. Metab. 57: 50.

Schenker JG, Polishuk WZ (1976b): An experimental model of ovarian hyperstimulation

syndrome. In: M Tischner, J Pilch, Krakow, Drukarnia Naukowa (eds.), Proceedings of the International Congress on Animal Reproduction, Vol. 4, p. 635.

Schenker JG, Schumert Z, Shifrin A, Spitz I (1977): Steroid pattern in experimental hyperstimulation syndrome and the response to indomethacin. Presented at the Second International Congress of Human Reproduction, Tel Aviv, October.

Schenker JG, Weinstein D (1978): Ovarian Hyperstimulation Syndrome: A Current Survey. Fertil. Steril. 30: 255.

Schieferstein G, Adam A, Armann J, Bantel E, Coerlin R, Egenrieder H, Fierlbeck G, Hook B, Schiek A, Schubring G, Schueer R (1987): Therapeutic results with tamoxifen in oligozoospermia: II. Hormonal analysis and semen parameters. Andrologia 19: 333.

Schill WB, Schumacher GFB (1973): Microradial diffusion in gel methods for the quantitative assessment of soluble proteins in genital secretions. In: RJ Blandau and K Moghissi (eds), The biology of the cervix. The University of Chicago Press, Chicago and London, pp. 173–200.

Schill WB, Braun-Falco O, Haberland GI (1974): The possible role of kinins in sperm motility. Intern. J. Fertil. 19: 163.

Schill WB (1975a): Caffeine and kallikrein induced stimulation of human sperm motility: A comparative study. Andrologia 7: 229.

Schill WB (1975b): Erste Ergebnisse einer parenteralen Behandlung von männlichen Fertilitätsstörungen mit Kallikrein: Oligozoospermie. Hautarzt 26: 541.

Schill WB, Landthaler M (1980): Tamoxifen treatment of olizoospermia. Andrologia 12: 546

Schill WB, Haberland GI (1975d): Wirkungen von verschiedenen Komponenten des Reninsystems auf die Spermatozoenmotilität in vitro. Klin. Wschr. 53: 73.

Schill WB (1986): Medical treatment of male infertility. In: V Insler, B Lunenfeld (eds.), Infertility – male and female. Churchill-Livingstone, London, p. 533.

Schirren CG (1972): Praktische Andrologie, Hartmann, Berlin.

Schlechte J, Vangilder J, Sherman B (1981): Predictors of the outcome of transphenoidal surgery for prolactin secreting pituitary adenomas. J. Clin. Endocrinol. Metab. 52: 785.

Schmidt SS (1975): Vas anastomosis: a return to simplicity. Brit. J. Urol. 47: 309.

Schmidt SS, Schoysman R, Stewart BH (1976): Surgical approaches to male infertility. In: ESE Hafez (ed.), Human semen and fertility regulation in man. Mosby, St. Louis, p. 476.

Schoemaker J, Simons AHM, Burger CW (1982): Induction of Ovulation with LH/FSH Releasing Hormone (LHRH). IVth Reinier de

Graaf Symposium. Excerpta Medica, Amsterdam 1982.

Schoenfeld C, Amelar RD, Dubin I (1975): Stimulation of ejaculated spermatozoa by caffeine. Fertil. Steril. 26: 158.

Schumacher GFB (1971): Soluble proteins in cervical secretions. In: AI Sherman, ChC Thomas (eds.), Pathways to conception, Springfield, Ill., pp. 168-187.

Schumacher GFB (1973a): Soluble proteins of human cervical mucus. In: M Elstein, K Moghissi and R Borth (eds.), Cervical mucus in human reproduction, Scriptor, Copenhagen, pp. 93-113.

Schumacher GFB (1973b): Soluble proteins in cervical mucus. In: RJ Blandau and K Moghissi (eds.), The biology of the cervix, University of Chicago Press, Chicago - London, p. 201.

Schwartz D, Laplance A, Jouannet P, David G (1979): Within subject variability of human semen with regard to sperm count, volume, total number of spermatozoa and length of abstinence. J. Reprod. Fert. 57: 391.

Schwarzel WC, Kruggel WG, Brodie HJ (1973): Studies on the mechanism of estrogen biosynthesis. VIII.: The development of inhibitors of the enzyme system in human placenta. Endocrinology 92: 866.

Scott LS, Young D (1962): Varicocele. Fertil. Steril. 13: 325.

Scott RS, Burger HG (1980): Inhibin is absent from azoospermic semen of infertile men. Nature 185: 246.

Scrabanek P, McDonald D, Meagher D, et al. (1980): Clinical course and outcome of 35 pregnancies in infertile hyperprolactinemic women. Fertil. Steril. 33: 391.

Seegar-Jones G, Moraes-Ruehsen MD (1967): Clomiphene citrate for improvement of ovarian function. Am. J. Obstet. Gynecol. 99: 814.

Seegar-Jones G, Maffezoli RQ, Rose GT, Kaplan G (1970): Pathophysiology of reproductive failure after clomiphene-induced ovulation. Am. J. Obstet. Gynecol. 108: 847-867.

Seegar-Jones GE, Acosta AA, Garcia JE, Rosenwaks Z (1985): Specific effects of FSH and LH on follicular development and oocyte retrieved as determined by a program for in vitro fertilization. Ann. New York Acad. Sci. 442: 119.

Seibel MM, Kamrava MM, McArdl C, Taymor ML (1984): Treatment of polycystic ovarian Disease with low-dose follicle stimulating hormone: Biochemical changes and ultrasound correlation. Int. J. Fertil. 29: 39-43.

Seidah NG, Arbatti NJ, Rochemont J, Sheth AR, Chretien M (1984): Complete amino acid sequence of human seminal plasma inhibin. FEBS, 175: 349.

Seki M, Tajima C, Maeda HR, Seki K, Yoshihara T (1973): Effect of quinestrol admini-

strated with clomiphene citrate on serum follicle-stimulating hormone and luteinizing hormone and other clinical findings. Am. J. Obstet. Gynecol. 116: 388-396.

Selin LK, Moger WH (1977): The effect of FSH on LH induced testosterone secretion in immature hypophysectomized male rats. Endocr. Res. Commun. 41: 171.

Serr DM, Ismajovich B (1963): Determination of the primary sex ratio for human abortions. Am. J. Obstet. Gynecol. 87: 63.

Serri O, Rasio E, Beauregard H et al. (1983): Recurrence of hyperprolactinemia after selective transsphenoidal adenomectomy in women with prolactinoma. N. Engl. J. Med. 309: 280.

Sertoli E (1865): Dell'esistenzia di particulari cellule ramifiate nei canalicoli seminiferi del testiculo umano. Il Morgagni 7: 31.

Setchell BP (1974a): Male fertility and sterility. Academic Press, London, New York, San Francisco.

Setchell BP (1974b): Secretions of the testis and epididymus. J. Reprod. Fert. 37:165.

Setchell BP, Jacks F (1974): Inhibition like activity in rat testis fluid. J. Endocr. 62: 675.

Settlage DS, Motoshimar M, Tredway R (1973): Sperm transport from the external cervical os to the fallopian tubes in women: a time and quantitation study. Fertil. Steril. 24: 655.

Shadmi A et al. (1987): Abolishment of the positive feedback mechanism: a criterion for temporary medical hypophysectomy by LHRH agonist. Gynecol. Endocrinol. 1: 1.

Shargil A (1987): Treatment of idiopathic hypogonadotropic hypogonadism in men with LHRH: A comparison of treatment with daily injections and with the pulsatile infusion pump. Fertil. Steril. 47: 492.

Sharpe RM, (1988): Endocrinology and paracrinology of the testes. In: Physiology and toxicology of male reproduction, edited by Lamb, J.C. IV. and Foster, P.M.D., San Diego, California: Academic Press, 1988, p. 71-99.

Sheikholislam BM, Stempfel RS Jr. (1972): Hereditary isolated somatotropin deficiency: Effects of human growth hormone administration. Pediatrics 49: 362.

Shelton RS, Van Campen MG Jr., Meisner DF et al. (1953): Synthetic estrogens: Halotriphenylethylene derivates. J. Am. Chem. Soc. 75: 5491.

Shepard MK, Balmaceda JP, Leija CG (1979): Relationship of weight to successful induction of ovulation with clomiphene citrate. Fertil. Steril. 32: 641.

Sher G, Knutzen VK, Stratton CJ, Montakhab MM, Allenson SG (1984): In vitro capacitation and transcervical intrauterine insemination for the treatment of refractory infertility: Phase I. Fertil. Steril. 41: 260.

Sheriff DS (1984): Hyperprolactinaemia and abnormal seminal cytology. In: W Thompson, RF Harrison, J Bonnar (eds), The male factor in human infertility. MTP Press Ltd, Lancaster Boston The Hague Dordrecht, 1984 p. 73.

Sherins RJ, Winters SJ, Wachslicht H (1977): Physiologic studies of the role of FSH in stimulation of spermatogenesis in the hypogonadotropic male. Symposium on: Recent progress in andrology. L'aquila, Italy, April 21-23 (Abstract).

Sherman JK (1986): Current status of cryobanking of human semen. In: JD Paulson, A Negro- Vilar, E Lucena, L Martini (eds), Andrology: Male Fertility and Sterility. Academic Press, New York, pp. 517.

Sheth AR, Mugtawada PP, Shah GV, Rao SS (1975): Occurence of prolactin in human semen. Fertil. Steril. 26: 905

Sheth AR, Vaze AY, Thakur AN (1978): Development of radioimmunoassay for inhibin. Ind. J. Exp. Biol. 16: 1025.

Shin SH (1982): Vasopressin has a direct effect on prolactin release in male rats. Neuroendocrinology 34: 55.

Shoham Z, Patel A, Jacobs HS (1991a): Polycystic ovarian syndrome: safety and effectiveness of stepwise and low-dose administration of purified follicle-stimulating hormone. Fertil. Steril. 55: 1051-1056.

Shome B, Parlow AF (1977): Human pituitary prolactin: The entire linear amino acid sequence. J. Clin. Endocrinol. Metab. 45: 1112.

Short RV (1974): Rhythms of ovulation. In: Chronobiological aspects of endocrinology. Symposia Medica Hoechst 9, FK Schattauer, pp. 221-228.

Shulman S (1972): Immunologic barriers to fertility. Obstet. and Gynec. Survey 27: 533-606.

Shulman GF, Shulman S (1982): Methylprednisolone treatment of immunologic infertility in the male. Fertil. Steril. 38: 591.

Sims JM (1869): Sperm penetration test on the microscope as an aid in the diagnosis and treatment of sterility. N.Y.J. Med. 8: 393.

Singer S, Sagiv M, Barnet M, Allalouf D, Landau B, Segereich E, Servadio C (1979): High sperm densities and the quality of semen. Arch. Androl. 3: 197.

Sinosich MJ, Lanzendorf SE, Hodgen GD (1989): Is microinjection the answer to male factor infertility? VI World Congress In Vitro Fertilization and Alternate Assisted Reproduction. Jerusalem, Israel April 2-7.

Skarin G, Nillius SJ, Wibell L, Wide L (1982): Chronic pulsatile low dose GnRH therapy for induction of testosterone production and spermatogenesis in a man with secondary hypogonadotropic hypogonadism. J. Clin. Endocrinol. Metab. 55: 723.

Skinner MK (1991): Cell-Cell interactions in the tesis. Endocrine Reviews 12: 45-77.

Skinner MK, Fritz IB (1985): Testicular peritubular cells secrete a protein under andro-gen control that modulates Sertoli cell function. Proc. Natl. Acad. Sci. USA 82: 114-118.

Skinner MK, Moses HL (1989): Transforming growth factor beta gene expression and action in the seminiferous tubule: peritubular cell-Sertoli cell interactions. Mol. Endocrinol. 3: 625.

Skinner MK, Takacs K, Coffey RJ (1989): Cellular localization of transforming growth factor-alpha gene expression and action in the seminiferous tubule: peritubular cell-Sertoli cell interactions. Endocrinology 124: 845.

Smals AG, Pieters GFF, Drayer JIM, Bernaad TJ, Kloppenberg PWC (1979): Leydig cell responsiveness to single and repeated human chorionic gonadotropin administration. J. Clin. Endocrinol. Metab. 49: 11.

Smith PE (1926): Hastening of development of female genital system by daily hemoplastic pituitary transplants. Proc. Soc. Exp. Biol. Med. 24: 131.

Smith PE, Engle ET (1927): Experimental evidence of the role of anterior pituitary in development and regulation of gonads. Am. J. Anatomy 40: 159.

Sobrero AJ, MacLead J (1962): The immediate postcoital test. Fertility and Sterility 13: 184-189.

Sobrero AJ (1974): Sperm migration in the human female. In: A Campos da Paz, T Hasegawa, Y Notake and M Hayashi (eds), Human reproduction, Igaki Shoin Ltd. Tokyo, pp. 47-53.

Sobrero AJ, Rehan NE (1975): The semen of fertile men. II. Semen characteristics of 1000 fertile men. Fertil. Steril. 26: 1048.

Sopelak VM, Hodgen GD (1984): Blockade of the estrogen induced luteinizing hormone surge in monkeys: a nonsteroidal, antigenic factor in porcine follicular fluid. Fertil. Steril. 41: 108-113.

Soloway M (1988): A phase III, multicenter comparison of depot zoladex and orchiectomy in patients with previously untreated, stage D-2 prostate cancer. Gynecological Endocrinology, 2 (Suppl. 1): 50.

Somazzi S, Goor W, Ott F (1973): The efficacy of various treatments in oligospermia. Dermatologia (Basel) 147/1: 37.

Southam AL, Janovsku NA (1962): Massive ovarian hyperstimulation with clomiphen citrate. J.A.M.A. 181: 443.

Spadoni LR, Cox DW, Smith DC (1974): Use of human menopausal gonadotropin for the induction of ovulation. Am. J. Obstet. Gynecol. 120: 988-993.

Spark RF, Pallotta J, Naftolin F, Clemens R (1976): Galactorrhea-amenorrhea syndromes: etiology and treatment. Ann. Intern. Med. 84 (5): 532-537.

Spellacy WN, Cohen WD (1967): Clomiphene treatment of prolonged secondary amenorrhea associated with pituitary gonadotropin deficiency. Am. J. Obstet. Gynecol. 97: 943–948.

Speroff L, Vande Wiele RL (1971): Regulation of the human menstrual cycle. Am. J. Obstet. Gynecol. 109: 234–247.

Steinberger E (1977): Male reproductive physiology. In: ATK Cockett, RL Urry (eds.), Male infertility, Grune and Stratton, New York – San Francisco – London, p. 1.

Steinberger E (1986): Pathophysiology of the testis. In: V Insler, B Lunenfeld (eds.), Infertility – Male and Female, Churchill Livingstone, Edinburgh – London – Melbourne – New York, p. 168.

Steinberger A, Elkington JSH, Sanborn BM, Steinberger E, Heindel JJ, Lindsey JN (1975): Culture and FSH responses of Sertoli cells isolated from sexually mature rat testis. In: Hormonal regulation of spermatogenesis. Plenum Press, p. 399.

Steinberger A, Herndel JJ, Lindsey JN, Elkington JSH, Sanborn BM, Steinberger E (1975): End. Res. Commu. 2: 261.

Steinberger A, Steinberger E (1976): Secretion of an FSH inhibiting factor by cultured Sertoli cells. Endocrinology 99: 918.

Stevenson AC, Johnson HA, Stewart PMI et al. (1966): Congenital malformations: a report of a study of a series of consecutive births in two centers. Bull. W.H.O. 34 (Suppl.) 9.

Stewart BH, Montie JE (1973): Male infertility: An optimistic report. J. Urol. 110: 216.

Sulewski JM, Eisenberg F, Slenger VG (1978): A longitudinal analysis of artificial insemination with donor semen. Fertil. Steril. 29: 524.

Sutherland RL (1981): Estrogen antagonists in chick oviduct: Antagonist activity of eight synthetic triphenylethylene derivatives and their interaction with cytoplasma and nuclear estrogen receptor. Endocrinology 109: 2061.

Swerdloff RS, Jacobs HS, Odell WP (1972): Role of synthetic progestagens in estrogen induction of LH and FSH surge. Endocrinology 90: 1529–1536.

Swyer GIM (1965): Clomiphene. In: CR Austin, JS Perry, E Churchill (eds.), Biol. Counc. Symp. on Aspects affecting Fertility. London, Churchill Davis, p. 180.

Swyer GIN, Radwanska E, McGarrigle HHG (1975): Plasma oestradiol and progesterone estimation for monitoring induction of ovulation with clomiphene and chorionic gonadotrophin. Br. J. Obstet. Gynaecol. 82: 794.

Syner FN, Moghissi KS (1971): Mucoids of cervical mucus. In: AI Sherman (ed.), Pathways to conceptions, Charles C Thomas Publisher, Springfield, Ill., pp. 156–167.

T

Tashjian AH Jr, Barowsky NJ, Jensen DK (1971): Thyrotropin releasing hormone: direct

evidence for stimulation of prolactin production by pituitary cells in culture. Biochem. Biophys. Res. Commun. 43: 516.

Thompson LR, Hansen LM (1970): Pergonal (menotropin): A summary of clinical experience in the induction of ovulation and pregnancy. Fertil. Steril. 21: 844–855.

Thorner MO, McNeilly AS, Hagan C, Besser GM (1974): Long-term treatment of galactorrhea and hypogonadism with bromocriptine. Br. Med. J. 2: 419–422.

Thorner MO, Besser GM, Jones A et al. (1975): Bromocriptine treatment of female infertility: report of 13 pregnancies. Br. Med. J. 4: 694.

Thorner MO, Besser GM (1977): Hyperprolactinemia and gonadal function: results of bromocriptine treatment. In: PG Crosignani, C Robyn (eds.), Prolactin and human reproduction. Academic Press, London, p. 285.

Thorner MO, Schran HF, Evans WS et al. (1980): A broad spectrum of prolactin suppression by bromocriptine in hyperprolactinemic women: a study of serum prolactin and bromocriptine levels after acute and chronic administration of bromocriptine. J. Clin. Endocrinol. Metab. 50: 1026.

Thorner MO, Perryman RL, Rogol AD et al. (1981): Rapid changes of prolactinoma volume after withdrawal and reinstitution of bromocriptine. J. Clin. Endocrinol. Metab. 53: 480.

Tietze Ch (1968): Fertility after discontinuation of intrauterine and oral contraception. Int. J. Fertil. 13: 385.

Toth A (1981): Abnormal seminal cytology in a patient with prolactin-secreting pituitary adenoma. Fertil. Steril. 27: 1425.

Tricomi V, Serr DM, Solish G (1960): The ratio of male and female embryos as determined by the sex chromatin. Am. J. Obstet. Gynecol. 75: 504.

Tsafriri A, Leiberman ME, Barnea A, Bauminger S, Lindner HR (1973): Induction by luteinizing hormone of ovum maturation and of steroidogenesis in isolated Graafian follicles of the rat: role of RNA and protein synthesis. Endocrinology 93: 1378–1386.

Tsapoulis AD, Zourlaz PA, Comninos AC (1978): Observations on 320 infertile patients treated with human gonadotropins (human menopausal gonadotropin/human chorionic gonadotropin). Fertil. Steril. 29: 492.

Tuang (1985): Personal communication to B. Lunenfeld.

Tulandi T, Micinnes RA, Arronet GH (1984): Ovarian hyperstimulation following ovulation induction with human menopausal gonadotropin. Int. J. Fertil. 29: 113.

Tulloch WS (1952): Consideration of sterility. Subfertility in the male. Edinburgh Med. J. 59: 29.

Tung PS, Fritz IB (1980): Interaction of Sertoli cells with myoid cells in vitro. Biol. reprod. 23: 207-217.

Turkalj I, Braun P, Krupp P (1982): Surveillance of bromocriptine in pregnancy. J.A.M.A. 247: 1589-1591.

Turner TT (1983): Varicocele: still an enigma. J. Urol. 129: 695.

U

Uehlig DT (1968): Fertility in men with varicocele. Int. J. Fertil. 13:58.

Urry RL (1977): Stress and infertility. In: ATK Cockett and RL Urry (eds.), Male infertility, Grune and Stratton, New York – San Francisco – London, p. 145.

Urry RL, Middleton RG, MacNamara L, Vikari CA (1983): The effect of single density bovine serum albumin columns on sperm concentration, motility and morphology. Fertil. Steril. 40: 666.

Vale W, Rivier J, Vaughan J, McClintock R, Corrigan A, Wood W, Karr D, Spiess D (1986): Purification and characterization of an FSH-releasing protein from porcine ovarian follicular fluid. Nature 321: 776.

Valk TW, Corley KP, Kelch RP, Marshal JC (1980): Hypogonadotropic hypogonadism: Hormonal responses to low dose pulsatile administration of gonadotropic releasing hormone. J. Clin. Endocrinol. Metab. 51: 730.

Valverde RC, Chieffo V, Reichlin S (1972): Prolactin releasing factor in porcine and rat hypothalamic tissue. Endocrinology 91: 982.

Van Beurden WMO, Roodnat B, De Jong FH, Muldere E, Van der Molen HJ (1976): Hormonal regulation of LH stimulation of testosterone production in isolated Leydig cells of immature rats: The effect of hypophysectomy, FSH, and estradiol–17B. Steroids 28: 847.

Vandenberg G, Yen SSC (1973): Effect of antiestrogenic action of clomiphene during the menstrual cycle: Evidence for a change in the feedback sensitivity. J. Clin. Endocrinol. Metab. 37: 356.

Van der Merwe JP, Kruger TF, Hulme VA et al. (1989a): Treatment of male sperm autoimmunity by GIFT with washed spermatozoa. Presented at the VI World Congress of In Vitro Fertilization and Alternative Assisted Reproduction, Jerusalem, Israel.

Van der Merwe JP, Kruger TF, Hulme VA et al. (1989b): Treatment of infertility due to teratozoospermia with GIFT. Presented at the VI World Congress of In Vitro Fertilization and Alternative Assisted Reproduction, Jerusalem, Israel.

Van der Molen HJ, Brinkman AO, Cooke BA, De Jong FH, Rommerts FFG, Van der Vusse GT (1972): The endocrine function of the human testis. Vol. I, Academic Press, London, New York.

Vaze AY, Thakur AN, Sheth AR (1980): Levels of inhibin in human semen and accessory reproductive organs. Andrologia 12: 66.

Verhoeven G, Cailleau J (1985): A factor in spent media from Sertoli cell-enriched cultures that stimulates steroidogenesis in Leydig cells. Mol. Cell. Endocrinol. 40: 57.

Vician L, Shupnik MA, Gorski J (1979): Effects of estrogen on primary bovine pituitary cell cultures: Stimulation of prolactin secretion, synthesis, and preprolactin messenger ribonucleic acid activity. Endocrinology 104: 736.

Videla E, Blanco AM, Galli ME, Fernandez-Collazo E (1981): Human seminal biochemistry: fructose, ascorbic acid, citric acid phosphatase and their relationship to sperm count. Andrologia 13: 212.

Vijayan E, McCann SM (1979): In vivo and in vitro effects of substance P and neurotensin on gonadotropin and prolactin release. Endocrinology 105: 64.

Virupannavar Ch, Tomera F (1982): An unusual case of retrograde ejaculation and a brief review of management. Fertil. Steril. 37: 275.

Votava Z, Lamplova I (1961): Antiserotonin activity of some ergolenyn and isoergolenyl derivatives in comparison with LSD and the influence of monoamine inhibition on this antiserotonin effect. In: E Rothlin (ed), Neuropsychotherapy (Vol. 2) Elsevier, Amsterdam, p. 68.

W

Wagenknecht LV, Klosterhalfen H, Schirren C (1980): Microsurgery in andrologic urology. I.: Refertilisation. J. Microsurg. 1: 370.

Wagenknecht LV (1982): Obstruction in the male reproductive tract. In: J Bain, WB Schill, L Schwarzstein (eds.), Treatment of male infertility. Springer-Verlag, Berlin – Heidelberg – New York, p. 221.

Wagner TOF, Brabant G, Von der Muehlen A (1985): Slow pulsing Oligospermia. In: TOF Brabant (ed.), Pulsatile LHRH therapy of the male. TM Verlag, Hameln, p. 111.

Wakeling AE, Visek WJ (1973): Insecticide inhibition of 5 dihydrotestosterone binding in the rat ventral prostrate. Science 181: 659.

Walsh PC, Swerdloff RS, Odell WD (1970): Cryptorchidism: effect on pituitary gonadotrophin secretion in the rat. Surg. Forum 21: 530.

Warner MP (1974): Artificial insemination, review after 32 years experience. NY State J. Med. 74: 2358.

Weber JM, Coelingh-Bennink HJT, Alsbach GPJ, Thyssen JHH (1983): The effect of pulsatile intravenous administration of LHRH on gonadotropin secretion in polycystic ovarian disease (Abstract). The 14th Acta Endocrinologica Congress, Stockholm, June 23-30.

Weed J, Carrera AE (1970): Glucose content of cervical mucus. Fertil. Steril. 21: 866-872.

Wehrenberg WB, McNicol D, Frantz AG, Ferin M (1980): The effects of serotonin on prolactin and growth hormone concentrations in normal and pituitary stalk-sectioned monkeys. Endocrinology 197: 1747–1750.

Weil C (1986): The safety of bromocriptine in long term use: a review of the literature. Curr. Med. Res. Opin. 10: 25–51.

Wetterauer U, Heite HJ (1980): Carnitine in seminal plasma: Its significance in diagnostic andrology. Arch. Androl. 4: 137.

Wildt I, Hausler A, Marshall G et al. (1981): Frequency and amplitude of gonadotropin-releasing hormone stimulation and gonadotropin secretion in the rhesus monkey. Endocrinology 109: 376.

Whitelaw MJ, Grams LR, Stamm WJ (1964): Clomiphene citrate: Its uses and observations on its probable action. Am. J. Obstet. Gynecol. 90: 355–363.

Whitelaw MJ, Kalman CE, Grams LR (1970): The significance of the high ovulation rate versus the low pregnancy rate with clomid. Am. J. Obstet. Gynecol. 107: 865–877.

Whitelaw MJ (1974): Observations on 1000 consecutive AID patients (Abstr.), 8th World Congress on Fertility and Sterility, Buenos Aires.

Whittaker PG, Wilcox T, Lind T (1981): Maintained fertility in a patient with hyperprolactinemia due to big, big prolactin. J. Clin. Endocrinol. Metab. 53: 863.

WHO Scientific Group Report. Agent stimulating gonadal function in the human. World Health Organization. Technical Report Series No. 514. WHO Consultation on the diagnosis and treatment of endocrine forms of female infertility (1976). B Lunenfeld (Chairman), J Jordan (Rapporteur), G Bettendorf, M Breckwoldt, E Del Pozo, V Insler, S Nillius, CA Pulsen, C Schirren, K Semm and WHO Secretariat: J Brarzelatto and J Spieler.

Wiebe RH, Hammond CB, Handwerger S (1977): Treatment of functional amenorrhea-galactorrhea with bromoergocryptine. Fertil-Steril. 28 (4): 426–433.

Williams RF, Hodgen GD (1980): Disparate effects of human chorionic gonadotropins during the late follicular phase in monkeys: Normal ovulation, follicular atresia, ovarian acyclicity and hypersecretion of follice-stimulating hormone. Fertil. Steril. 33: 64.

Winters SJ (1990): Inhibin is released together with testosterone by the human testis. J. Clin. Endocrinol. Metab. 70: 548.

Wright WW, Frenkel AI (1980): An androgen receptor in the nuclei of late spermatid in testes of male rats. Endocrinology 107: 314.

Wu C (1977): Plasma hormones in human gonadotropin induced ovulation. Obstet. Gynecol. 49: 308.

Y

Yaoi Y, Bettendorf G (1973): Effects of retroprogesterone, clomid and sexovid on gonadotropin release in rats. In: T Hagesgawa, M Hayashi, FJG Ebling, IW Henderson (eds.), Fertility and sterility, Excerpta Medica, Amsterdam, pp. 638–639.

Yen SSC (1983): Clinical applications of gonadotropin-releasing hormone and gonadotropin-releasing hormone analogs. Fertil. Steril. 39: 257.

Younglai EV (1975): Steroid production by the isolated rabbit ovarian follicle. III.: Actinomycin D – intensive stimulation of steroidogenesis by LH. Endocrinology 96: 468–474.

Z

Zaneveld LJD, Polakoski KL (1977): Collection and physical examination of the ejaculate. In: ESE Hafez (ed.), Techniques of human andrology. Elsevier, North Holland, Amsterdam – New York – Oxford, p. 147.

Zondek B (1926a): Über die Funktion des Ovarium. Dtsch. Med. Wsch. 18: 343.

Zondek B (1926b): Über die Funktion des Ovarium. Z. Geburtsh. Gynäk. 90: 372.

Zrubek H, Czajka R, Lopucka M (1986): Estimation of effectiveness of epimestrol (Stimovul) therapy in treatment of anovulatory cycles in sterile women of the IInd Group according to WHO. In: TE Soon, SS Ratnam, LS Min (eds.), 12th World Congress on Fertility and Sterility, Singapore, 1986, p. 110.

Zuckerman Z, Rodriguez Rigau LJ, Smith KD, Steinberger E (1977): Frequency distribution of sperm counts in fertile and infertile males. Fertil. Steril. 28: 1310.

List of Terms